I0783194

THE JOURNEY TO MASTERING MASSAGE

A Step-by-Step Guide to Techniques for Relaxation, Pain Relief and Stress Management

Copyright © 2024 by Nicholas K. N.

All rights reserved. No part of this book may be copied, distributed, or transmitted in any form or by any means, including photocopying, recording, or other electronic or mechanical methods, without prior written permission from the publisher, except for brief quotations used in reviews or educational discussions.

For permissions or inquiries, contact:
nmwakuni@gmail.com

Disclaimer: This book is intended for educational purposes only. Always consult a licensed professional for medical advice or treatment.

Dedication

For the caregivers, the healers, and those who bring light into the lives of others. Your touch changes the world.

Acknowledgments

Writing this book has been a journey of learning, growth, and collaboration. I am deeply grateful to Harrison Mwakuni. Thank you for your guidance, inspiration, and support.

Special thanks to Evans Howard for your invaluable feedback and encouragement, and to my family and friends for their unwavering belief in this project.

TABLE OF CONTENTS

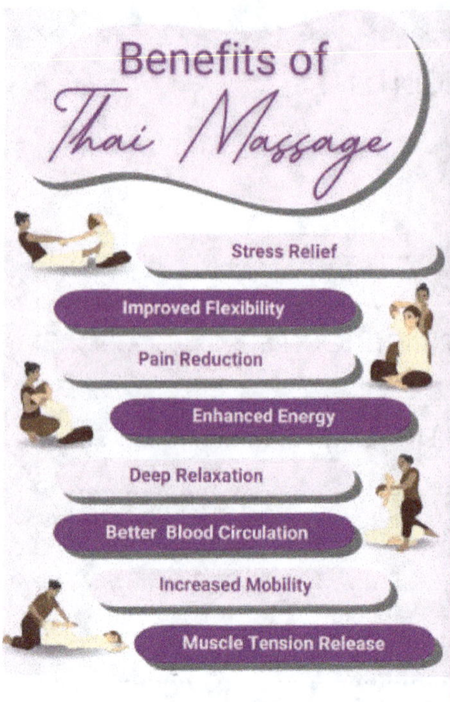

Benefits of
Thai Massage
Stress Relief
Improved Flexibility
Pain Reduction
Enhanced Energy
Deep Relaxation
Better Blood Circulation
Increased Mobility
Muscle Tension Release

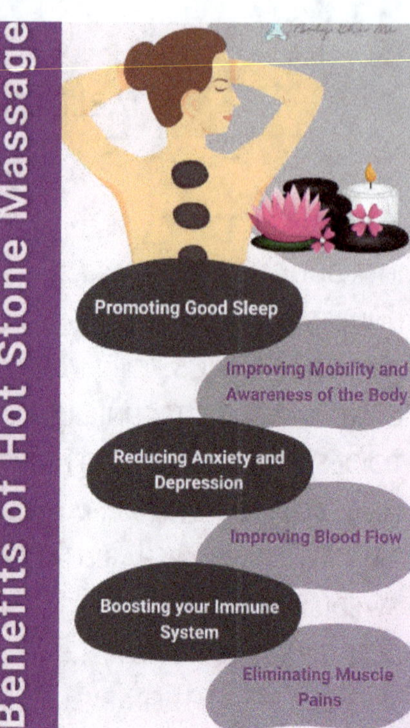

Benefits of Hot Stone Massage
Promoting Good Sleep
Improving Mobility and Awareness of the Body
Reducing Anxiety and Depression
Improving Blood Flow
Boosting your Immune System
Eliminating Muscle Pains

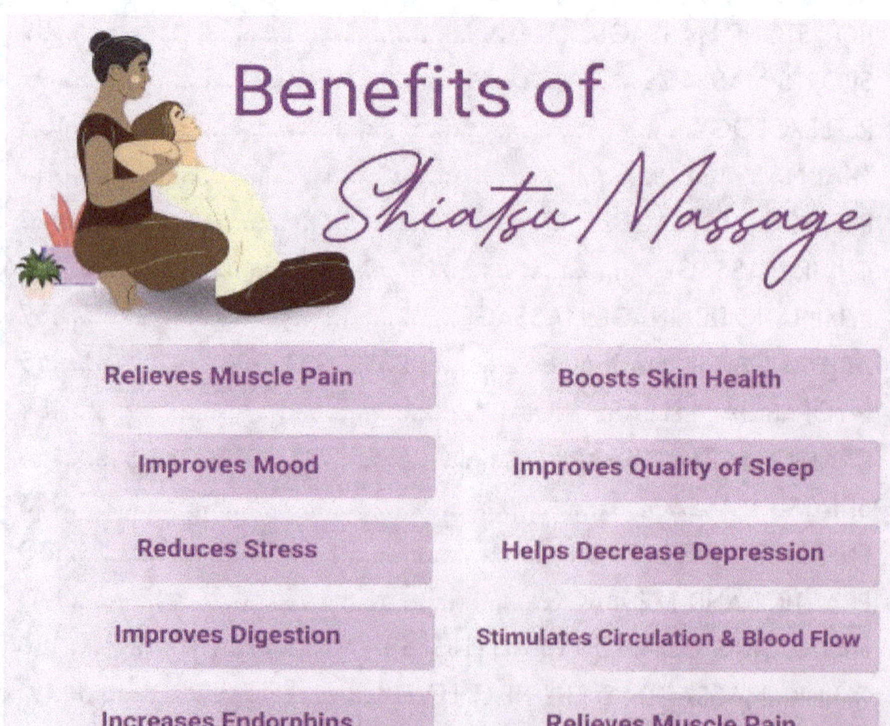

Benefits of
Shiatsu Massage
Relieves Muscle Pain
Boosts Skin Health
Improves Mood
Improves Quality of Sleep
Reduces Stress
Helps Decrease Depression
Improves Digestion
Stimulates Circulation & Blood Flow
Increases Endorphins
Relieves Muscle Pain

INTRODUCTION

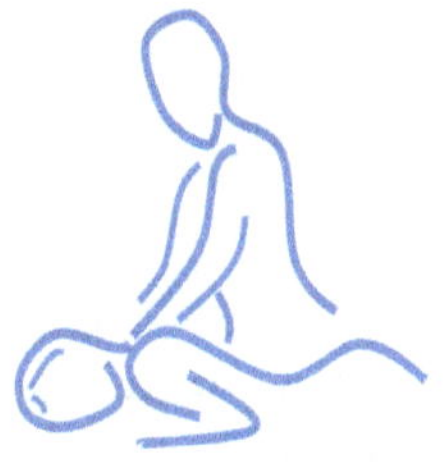

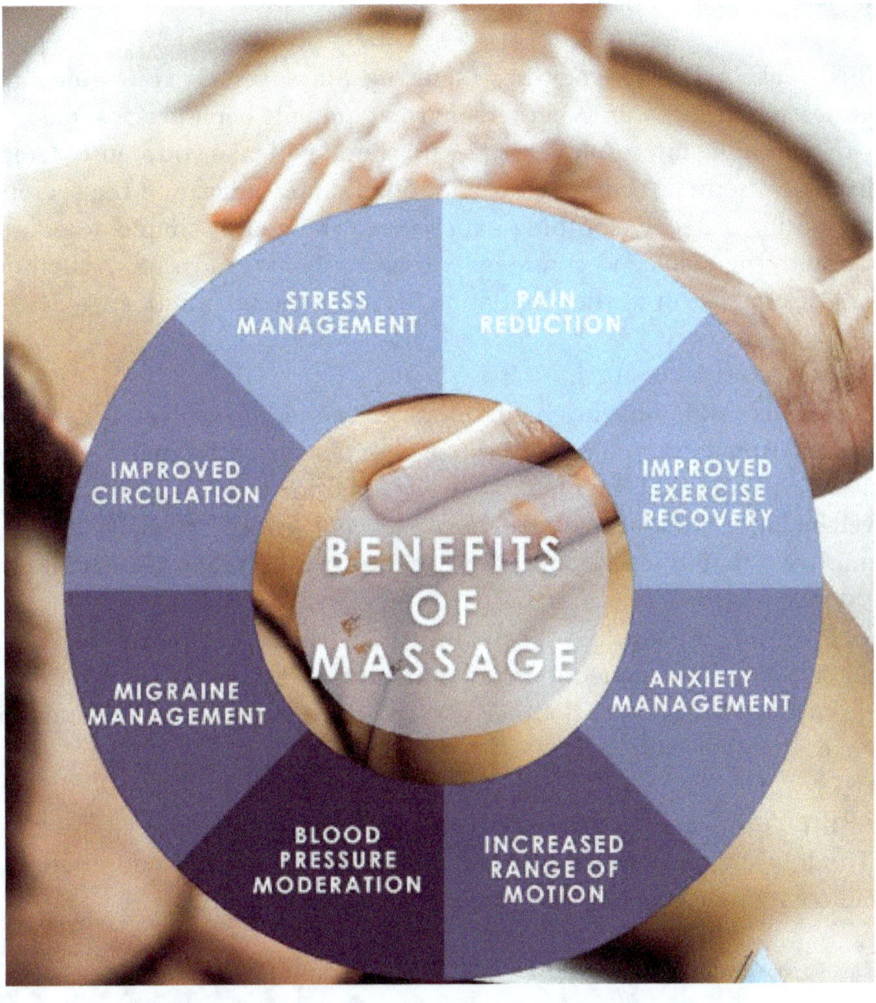

Imagine coming home after a long day, your body tense and your mind racing. Someone places their hands gently on your shoulders, applying just the right amount of pressure, and suddenly, the weight of the day begins to lift. That is the power of massage—a timeless practice that transcends cultures and generations to bring relief, healing, and connection.

Massage is more than just a series of techniques. It is an art and a science rooted in the simple yet profound act of touch. Over the centuries, people have used massage not only to alleviate physical discomfort but also to foster emotional well-being and even deepen personal relationships. In today's fast-paced world, where stress and physical strain are constants, massage remains as relevant as ever, offering a pathway to relaxation, recovery, and rejuvenation.

This book, " **The Journey to Mastering Massage,**" is your guide to harnessing that power. Whether you're a complete beginner or someone with a budding interest in massage, this book will take you step-by-step through essential techniques, foundational knowledge, and the secrets to creating a deeply soothing experience. The goal is simple: to equip you with the skills and confidence to give effective massages, whether for personal use or as the foundation for professional practice.

Why Learn Massage?

Massage is a skill that enriches both the giver and the receiver. When you massage someone, you're not just easing their physical tension—you're also contributing to their mental clarity, emotional balance, and overall well-being. Studies show that massage can reduce stress hormones, improve circulation, enhance sleep quality, and even boost the immune system.

For the giver, massage is a deeply rewarding practice. It fosters empathy, builds a sense of connection, and cultivates mindfulness. It's a chance to slow down, tune into another person's needs, and use your hands to make a tangible difference.

What You'll Learn in This Book

"The Journey to Mastering Massage" is designed to be clear, practical, and comprehensive. Here's what you can expect to find:

Core Techniques: You'll learn the fundamental strokes and movements that form the backbone of effective massage therapy, including how to adjust pressure and rhythm to suit individual needs.

Understanding the Body: Gain insights into the anatomy of key muscle groups and how massage affects the body's systems, such as circulation and the nervous system.

Creating the Right Environment: Learn how to set the stage for a relaxing and effective massage, including tips on lighting, tools, and ambiance.

Targeted Approaches: Explore specific techniques for managing stress, alleviating pain, and supporting recovery from injuries or intense physical activity.

Practical Applications: Discover how to give massages at home, on loved ones, or in a professional setting, with step-by-step instructions tailored for various scenarios.

A Skill for Life

The beauty of massage is its versatility. It can be a quick remedy for a loved one's headache or a full-body session to help someone recover from a tough week. Whatever your motivation, the skills you develop will stay with you, ready to use whenever the opportunity arises.

As you embark on this journey, remember that mastery doesn't happen overnight. Like any art, massage requires patience, practice, and a willingness to learn. But with every session, you'll grow more confident in your ability to provide comfort, ease tension, and foster connection.

So, let's begin this journey together. By the end of this book, you'll not only have the knowledge to perform a great massage—you'll also have the tools to make a meaningful difference in the lives of those you touch.

Welcome to the world of healing hands. Let's get started.

Diag: Body Muscles

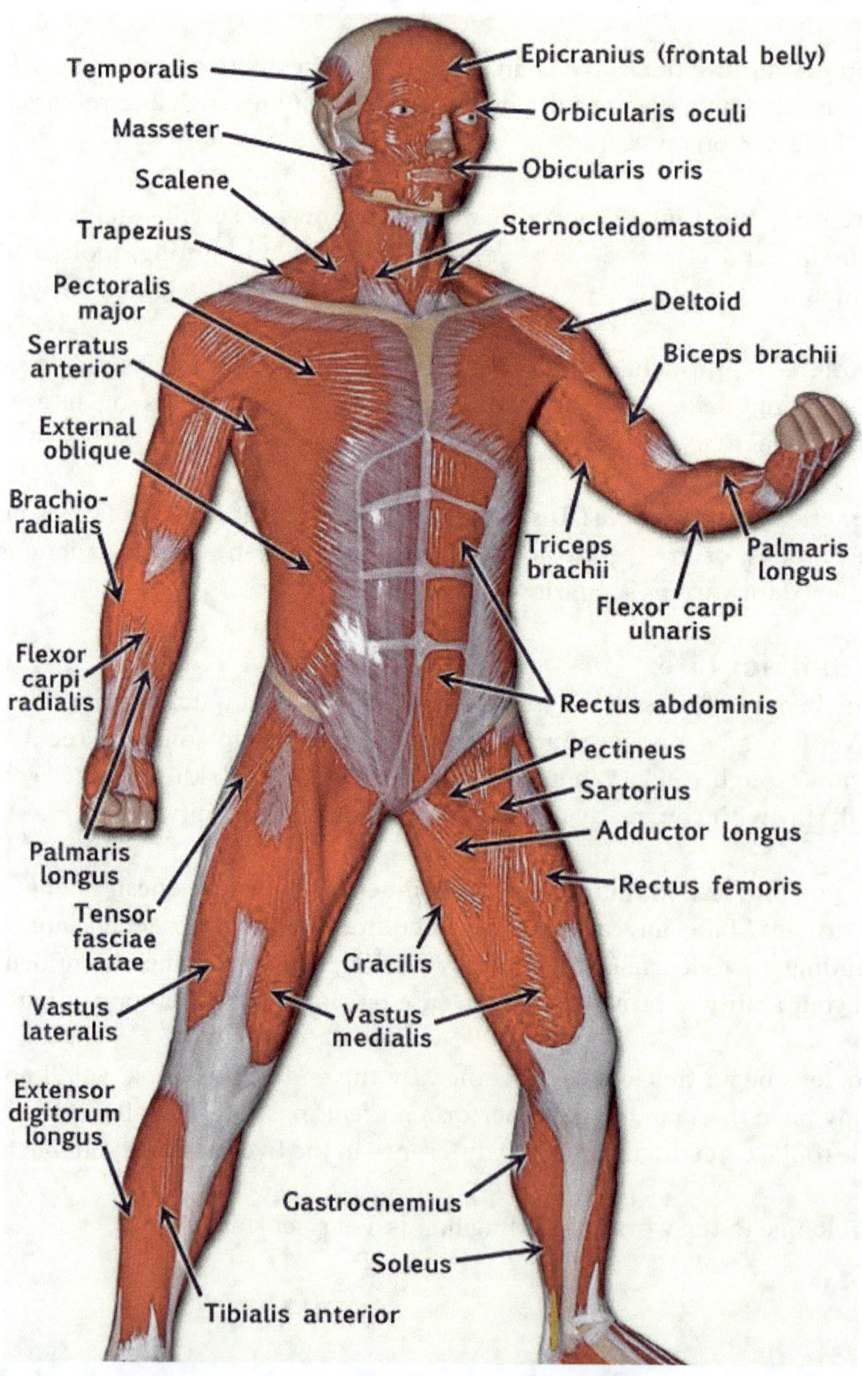

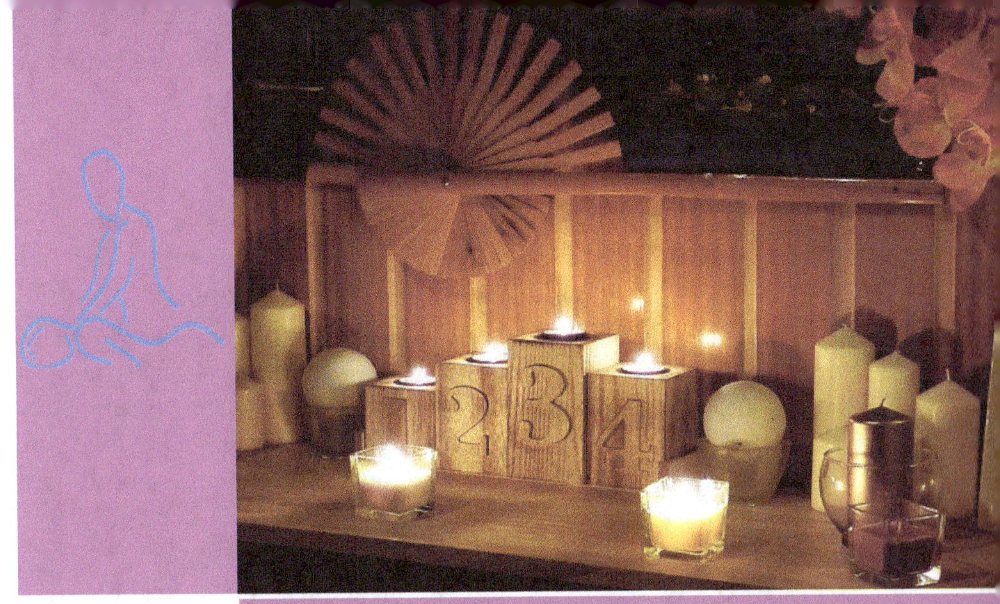

1

UNDERSTANDING MASSAGE THERAPY

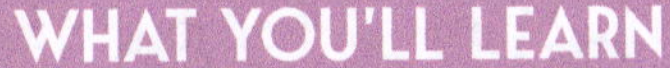

WHAT YOU'LL LEARN

◊ CORE PRINCIPLES AND PHILOSOPHY OF MASSAGE

◊ TYPES OF MASSAGE

◊ BENEFITS OF MASSAGE

The Foundation of Healing Touch

Massage therapy is not just about relieving muscle soreness or indulging in a pampering session. It is a time-honored healing practice that touches upon both the physical and emotional aspects of health. From its roots in ancient cultures to its modern-day popularity, massage has evolved into a sophisticated and diverse method of promoting overall wellness. Whether you seek relief from chronic pain, the benefits of stress reduction, or an overall sense of balance and relaxation, massage therapy offers a unique way to nurture both your body and mind.

In this chapter, we will delve into the principles and philosophy that form the foundation of massage therapy, explore the different types of massage techniques, and uncover the physical, emotional, and mental benefits that massage offers. Whether you're new to the practice or looking to deepen your understanding, this chapter will provide essential insights that will guide you on your journey to wellness through the power of touch.

The Core Principles and Philosophy of Massage Therapy

Massage therapy operates on the premise that the body, mind, and spirit are interconnected, and true healing happens when these elements are brought into harmony. While this may seem like an ancient or spiritual idea, it's also rooted in physiological principles that we now understand scientifically. When we experience stress, anxiety, or physical pain, it often manifests as tension in the muscles, tightness in the body, or a disruption of our emotional state. Massage is a way to alleviate these physical symptoms while promoting mental and emotional healing.

Holistic Healing:

At the heart of massage therapy is the holistic philosophy, which is based on the understanding that the body should be treated as a whole, rather than as separate, isolated parts. This means that massage therapy addresses not only physical discomfort but also emotional and psychological imbalances that may be contributing to the problem. For example, someone suffering from chronic lower back pain may also be experiencing emotional stress that has compounded the physical discomfort. By addressing both aspects—through massage techniques that release muscular tension and through creating an environment of emotional safety—massage therapy seeks to restore overall balance. Massage's holistic approach also involves recognizing how various systems in the body (nervous, muscular, circulatory, and lymphatic) are interconnected. A blockage in one system can cause problems in another, and massage helps move energy and fluids through the body, facilitating healing. This is why massage is effective for people with a wide range of issues, from muscle pain to digestive issues, anxiety, and even sleep disorders.

The Power of Touch:

Touch is one of the most fundamental and ancient forms of healing. In fact, human touch has been shown to reduce stress, lower blood pressure, and improve the immune system's function. When performed mindfully, massage is more than just a physical treatment; it is a therapeutic, nurturing interaction that promotes a sense of comfort and well-being. Touch activates receptors in the skin that send messages to the brain, which in turn releases endorphins, dopamine, and serotonin—chemicals that promote feelings of happiness, relaxation, and well-being. These biochemicals contribute to the reduction of pain, alleviation of stress, and improvement of mood.

Massage therapists are highly attuned to the power of touch and use their skills to communicate with the body in a way that helps release tension, pain, and emotional blockages. This form of non-verbal communication allows therapists to provide healing to clients who may not have the words to express their discomfort or emotional stress.

Personalized Care

One of the most remarkable aspects of massage therapy is its ability to adapt to the needs of each individual. While the techniques themselves may be standardized, massage therapy is a personalized practice. Every person's body is different, and massage therapists adjust their approach based on the client's physical condition, comfort level, and emotional needs.

A skilled therapist will assess the client's posture, muscle tightness, and movement patterns to determine which techniques to apply. This individualized approach ensures that the client receives the maximum benefit from the session. A deeper, firmer technique might be used on someone with chronic muscle stiffness, while a gentler approach might be more appropriate for someone seeking relaxation and stress relief.

Types of Massage

Massage therapy is not a single, uniform practice. There are numerous styles and techniques, each with its own set of benefits and applications. From Swedish massage to specialized treatments like aromatherapy or deep tissue therapy, there is something for everyone. Let's explore some of the most commonly used types of massage:

1. Swedish Massage

Often considered the classic form of massage, Swedish massage is ideal for those who are new to massage or simply looking to relax. It involves a series of long, fluid strokes that are designed to increase circulation, reduce muscle tension, and enhance relaxation. The therapist may also use kneading, tapping, and friction to reach deeper layers of muscle tissue. Swedish massage is gentle and soothing, making it a popular choice for individuals who seek a calming experience rather than pain relief. It also has a variety of health benefits, including stress reduction and improved flexibility. For this massage, the recipient removes their clothes, though they may choose to keep their underwear on. They'll be covered with a sheet while lying on the massage table. The massage therapist will move the sheet to uncover areas that they are actively working on. Usually, a Swedish massage will last 60 to 90 minutes.

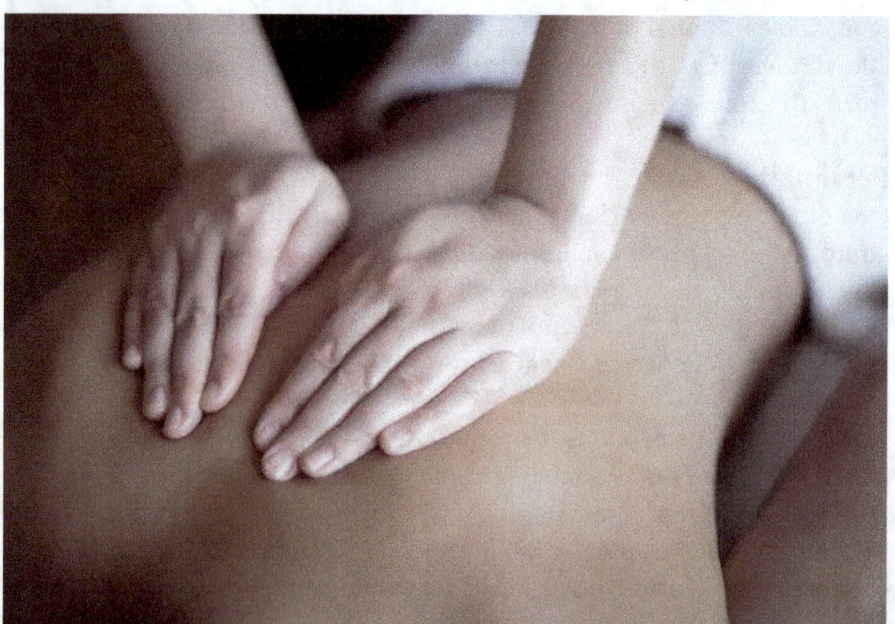

2. Deep Tissue Massage

While Swedish massage is all about relaxation, deep tissue massage targets the deeper layers of muscle tissue and fascia. This technique uses firm pressure and slow, deliberate strokes to break down chronic muscle tension and release stubborn knots. Deep tissue massage is particularly helpful for individuals with long-term muscle stiffness, lower back pain, or those recovering from injuries. It's an excellent way to improve mobility and relieve chronic discomfort, although it may cause some discomfort during the session, especially in areas with significant muscle tension.The recipient can be naked during this massage or wear their underwear. The massage will last 60 to 90 minutes. While deep tissue may be more intense, the recipient shouldn't feel any pain or soreness.

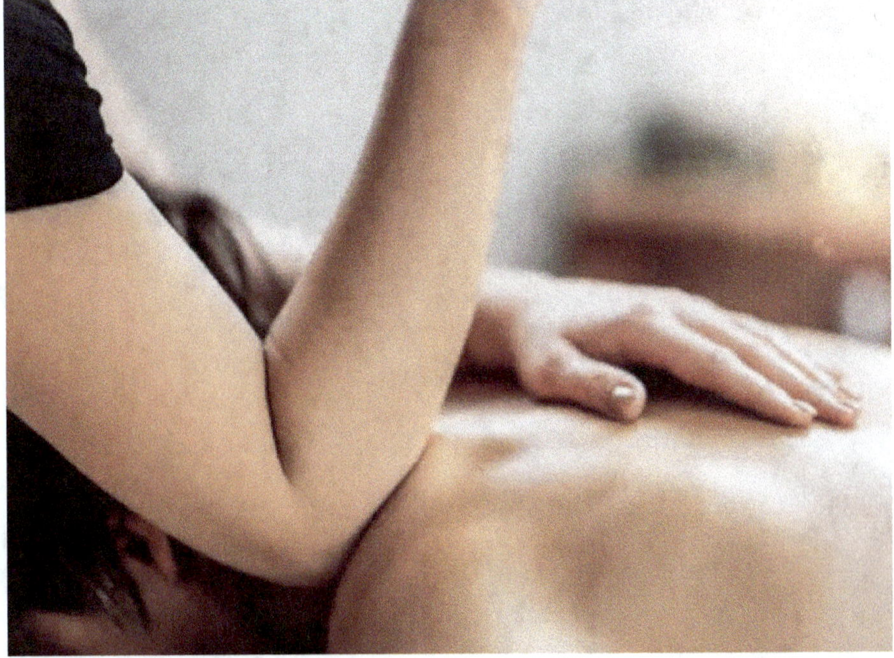

3. Trigger Point Therapy

Trigger points are areas of intense muscle tightness that can refer pain to other areas of the body. For example, a tight knot in the shoulder might radiate pain into the neck or down the arm. Trigger point therapy is a technique used to apply concentrated pressure to these points to relieve pain and discomfort. By targeting specific spots, this therapy can help break down muscle tension, improve circulation, and restore proper function to the muscles. It's especially helpful for individuals suffering from chronic pain or specific, localized muscle issues, such as tension headaches, sciatica, or myofascial pain syndrome. The massage will include work on the entire body, though the therapist will focus on specific areas that need to be released. The recipient can wear lightweight clothing for the massage, or they can be fully or partially undressed. This type of massage will usually last 60 to 90 minutes.

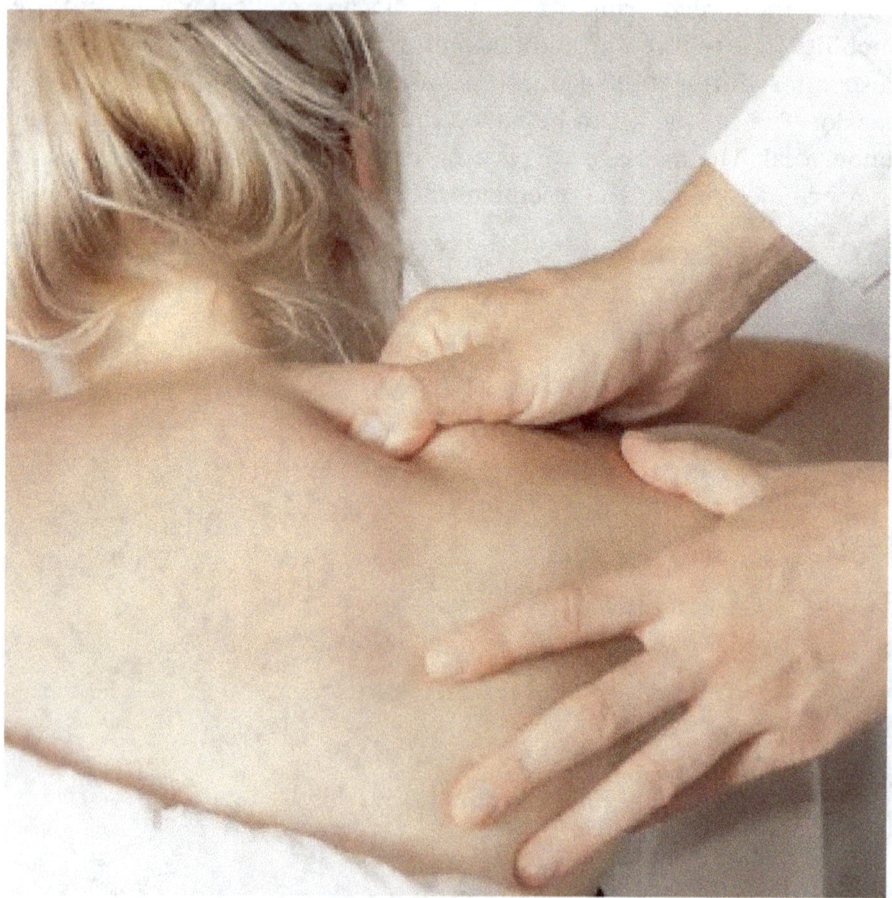

4. Aromatherapy Massage

Aromatherapy massage blends the therapeutic benefits of essential oils with the art of massage. The therapist selects oils based on the client's specific needs, whether it's calming lavender for relaxation or invigorating eucalyptus for energy. These essential oils are often inhaled during the session, allowing the aromatic molecules to stimulate the olfactory system, which can trigger emotional and psychological responses. Aromatherapy massage is ideal for those seeking to address emotional issues, such as anxiety, insomnia, or stress, while also benefiting from the relaxing effects of massage. The recipient won't wear any clothing, but underwear is optional. An aromatherapy massage is 60 to 90 minutes.

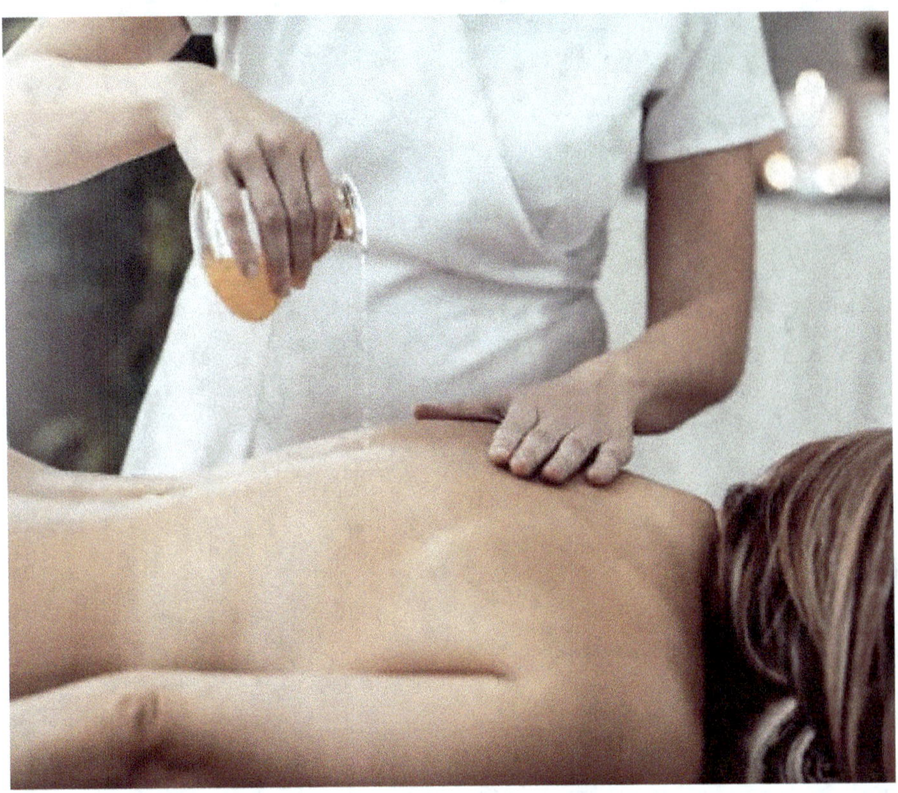

5. Hot Stone Massage

In hot stone massage, the therapist uses smooth, heated stones placed along the body to promote deep muscle relaxation. The warmth of the stones helps increase blood flow, melt away muscle tension, and reduce pain. The therapist may also use the stones to apply gentle pressure during the massage. This technique is particularly beneficial for people with chronic pain, muscle stiffness, or those simply seeking a deeply relaxing experience. The use of heat combined with the therapist's touch creates a soothing experience that enhances relaxation and promotes a sense of calm. Recipients don't wear clothes for a hot stone massage, unless they'd prefer to wear their underwear. They'll be covered with a sheet. Usually, the massage is 90 minutes long.

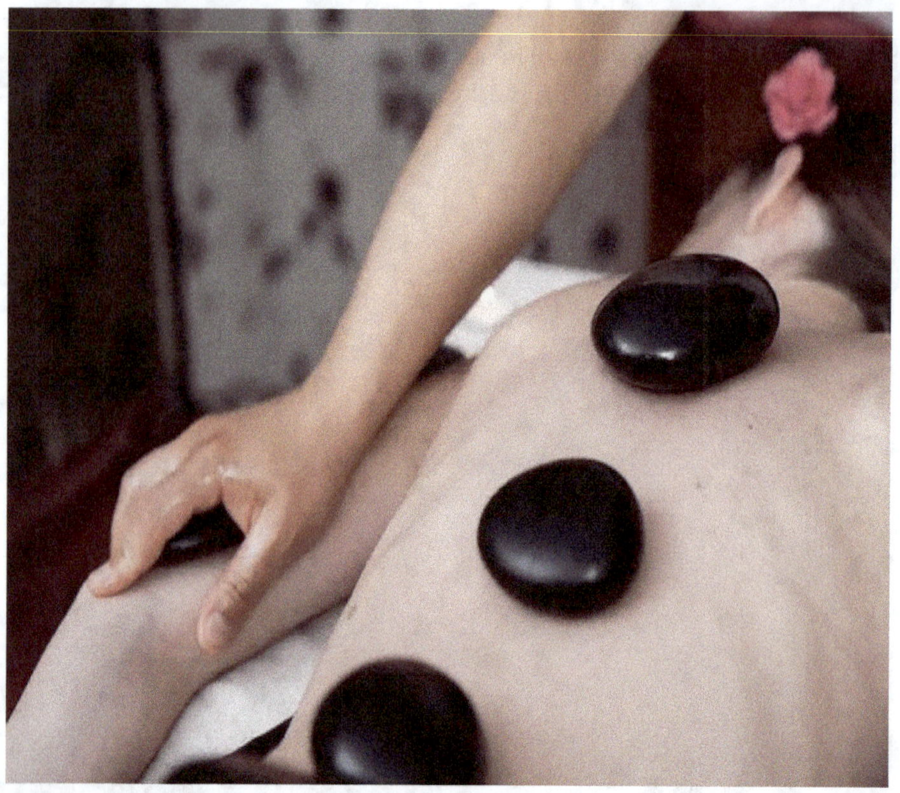

6. Shiatsu Massage

Shiatsu is a Japanese technique that uses finger pressure along the body's energy pathways, called meridians. It is based on the principles of Traditional Chinese Medicine and aims to restore balance to the body's energy flow. Shiatsu works by applying rhythmic pressure to specific points along the meridians, much like acupressure, to release blockages and improve overall health. This type of massage is especially beneficial for people looking to address energy imbalances, boost vitality, or reduce stress. It can be done with the client fully clothed, making it a more accessible option for those who prefer not to undress during the session. Shiatsu massages typically last 60 to 90 minutes.

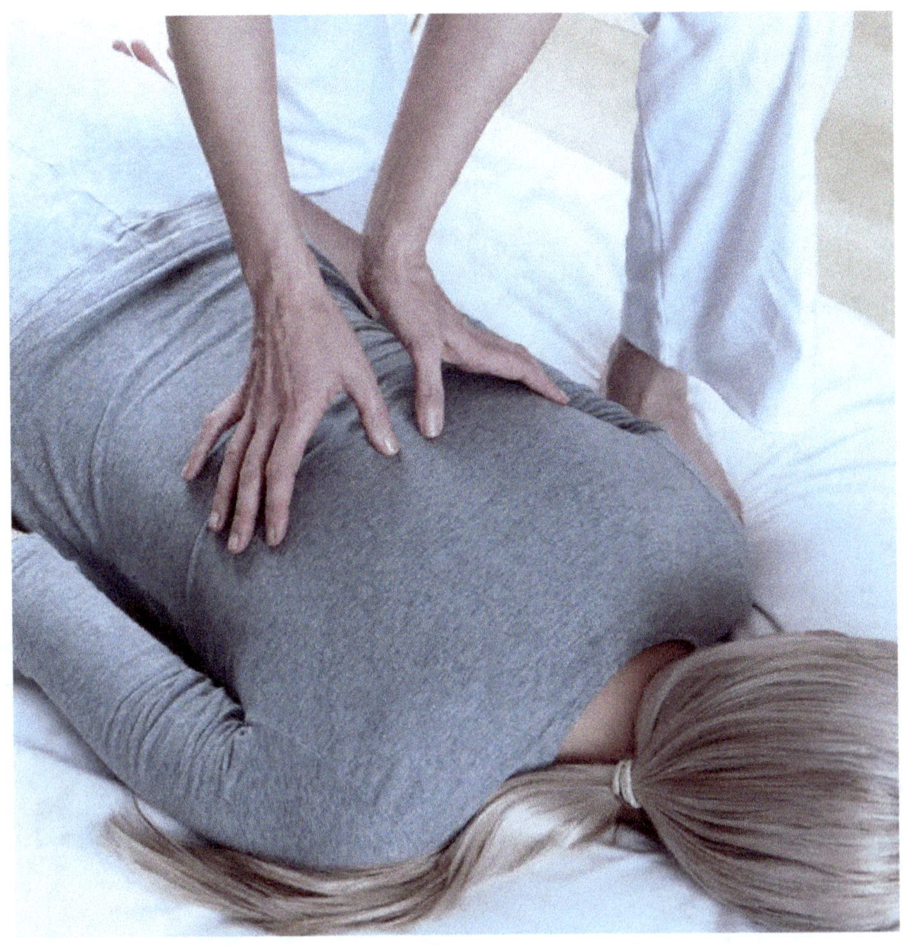

7. Sports Massage

Designed specifically for athletes or physically active individuals, sports massage is tailored to prevent injuries, improve performance, and enhance recovery. It involves a combination of techniques, including deep tissue, stretching, and friction, to target overworked muscles and reduce the risk of injury. Whether before an event, after an event, or as part of a regular training routine, sports massage helps keep muscles flexible, promote healing, and reduce fatigue. This type of massage is ideal for athletes or anyone who engages in physical activity on a regular basis. One can have a sports massage while clothed or naked. If they prefer to wear clothing then it should be loose, allowing the therapist to access their muscles. Loose shorts and a tank top are options. The massage will likely last 60 to 90 minutes.

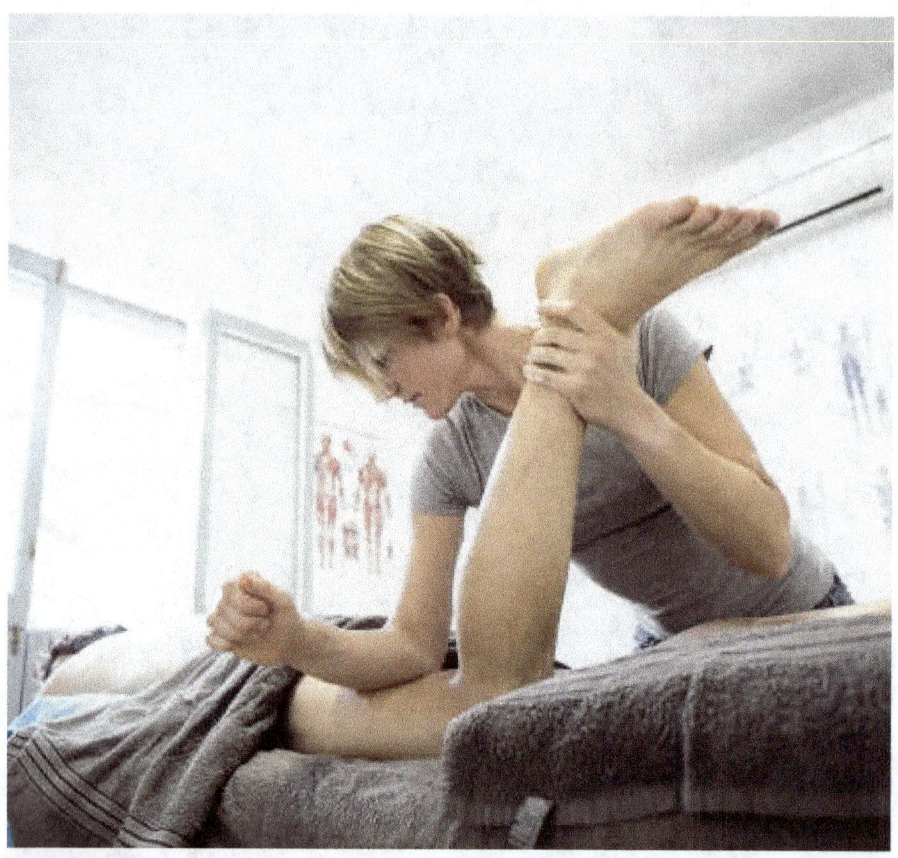

8. Reflexology

Reflexology uses gentle to firm pressure on different pressure points of the feet, hands, and ears. It's best for people who are looking to relax or restore their natural energy levels. It's also a good option for those who aren't comfortable being touched on the entire body. Reflexology may be especially beneficial for relaxation, reduced pain, reduced fatigue, improved sleep, reduced anxiety and improved mood. One can wear loose, comfortable clothing that allows access to their legs. A reflexology massage lasts 30 to 60 minutes.

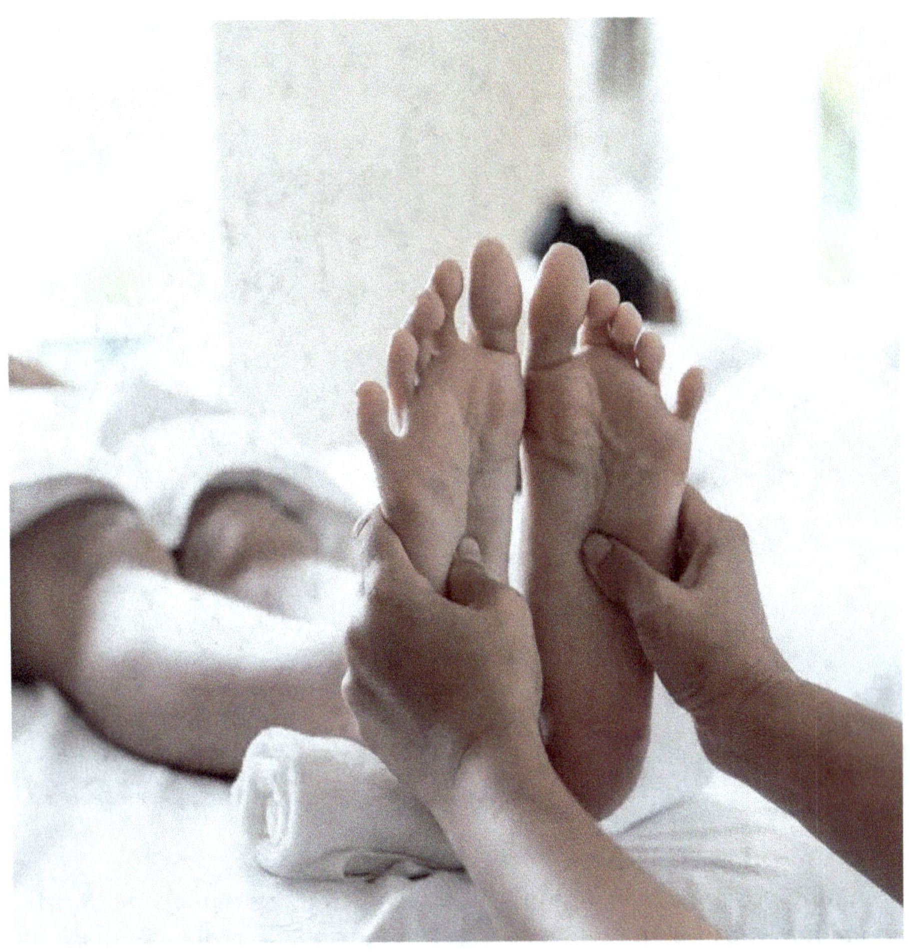

9. Thai massage

Thai massage is best for people who want a more active form of massage and want to reduce and relieve pain and stress. It can also help improve flexibility, circulation and energy levels. Thai massage works the entire body using a sequence of movements that are similar to yogic stretching. Your therapist will use their palms and fingers to apply firm pressure to your body. You'll also be stretched and twisted into various positions. One can wear loose, comfortable clothing during the massage. A Thai massage lasts 60 to 90 minutes.

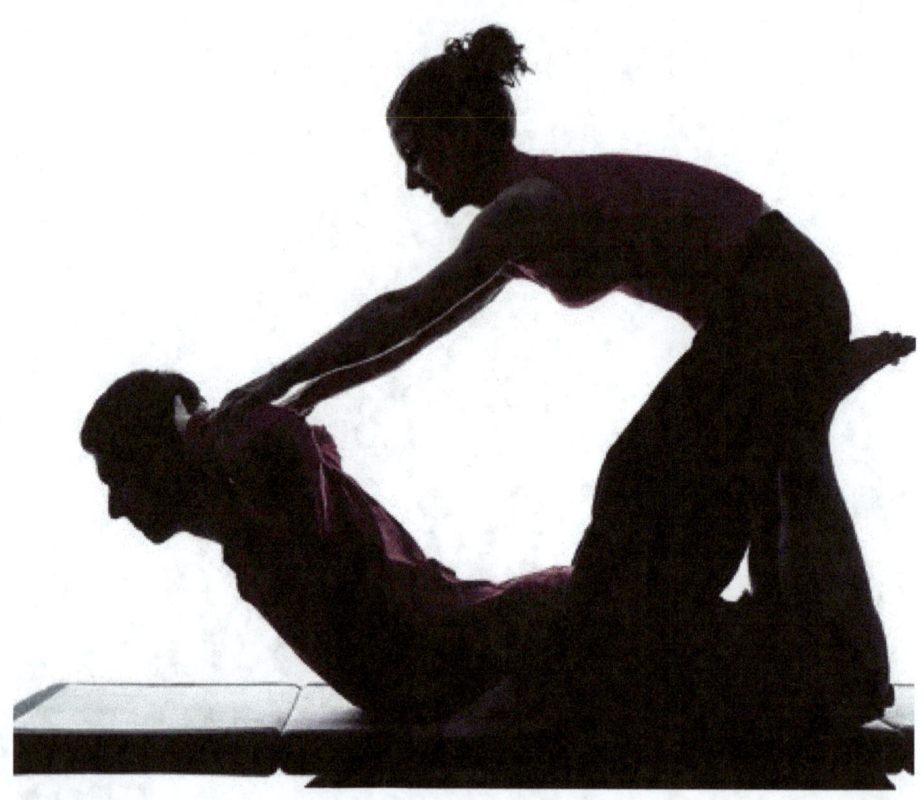

10. Prenatal massage

Prenatal massage can be a safe way for women to get a massage during pregnancy. It can help reduce pregnancy body aches, reduce stress, and ease muscle tension. However, many facilities, especially in the United States, do not offer massages to women in their first trimester due to the risk of miscarriage during this time. Prenatal massage uses mild pressure similar to Swedish massage. The therapist will focus on areas such as your lower back, hips, and legs. The recipient can be fully or partially undressed, depending on their comfort level. During the massage, they'll either lie on their side or on a specially designed table with a cutout for your belly. The massage will usually last 45 to 60 minutes.

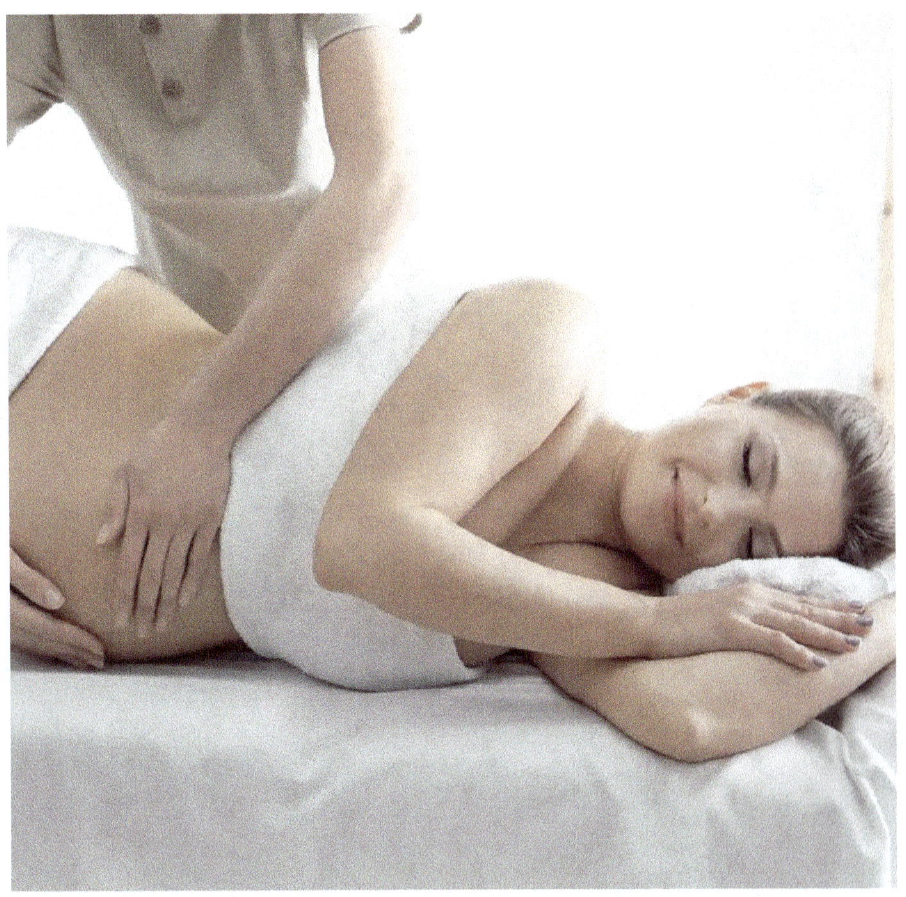

11. Chair massage

A chair massage is best for people who want a quick massage that focuses on the neck, shoulders, and back. A chair massage can be a comfortable introduction to massage if you've never had one before. A Chair massage also helps relieve stress and promote relaxation. This type of massage uses light to medium pressure. During the massage, the recipients remain fully clothed and sit in a specially designed chair. They'll straddle the chair so that their chest pushes into the back of the chair, allowing the massage therapist to have access to your back. These massages are usually 10 to 30 minutes.

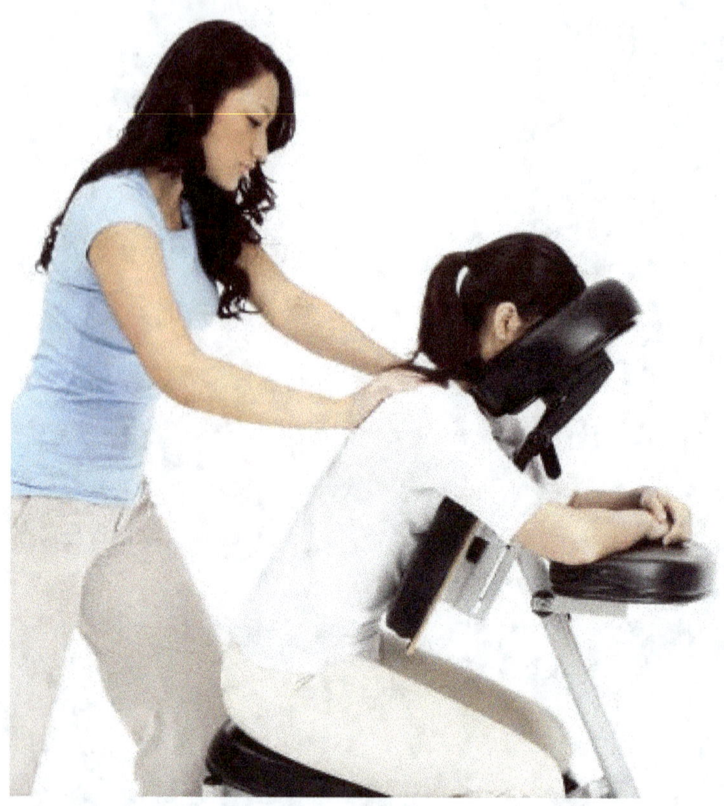

12. Lymphatic drainage massage

Lymphatic drainage massage, also known as manual lymphatic drainage (MLD), is a type of gentle massage that encourages the lymph fluids to circulate through the body. The lymphatic system helps remove toxins, and improved circulation can help with a number of conditions, including lymphedema, insomnia, edema, skin disorders, fatigue, stress, digestive problems, arthritis and migraines.

One shouldn't receive lymphatic drainage massage if they have any of the following conditions:

- congestive heart failure

- history of blood clots or stroke

- current infection

- liver problems

- kidney problems

It's possible to perform lymphatic drainage massage on yourself at home. Alternatively, one can seek out a professional. These massages usually last 60 minutes or longer.

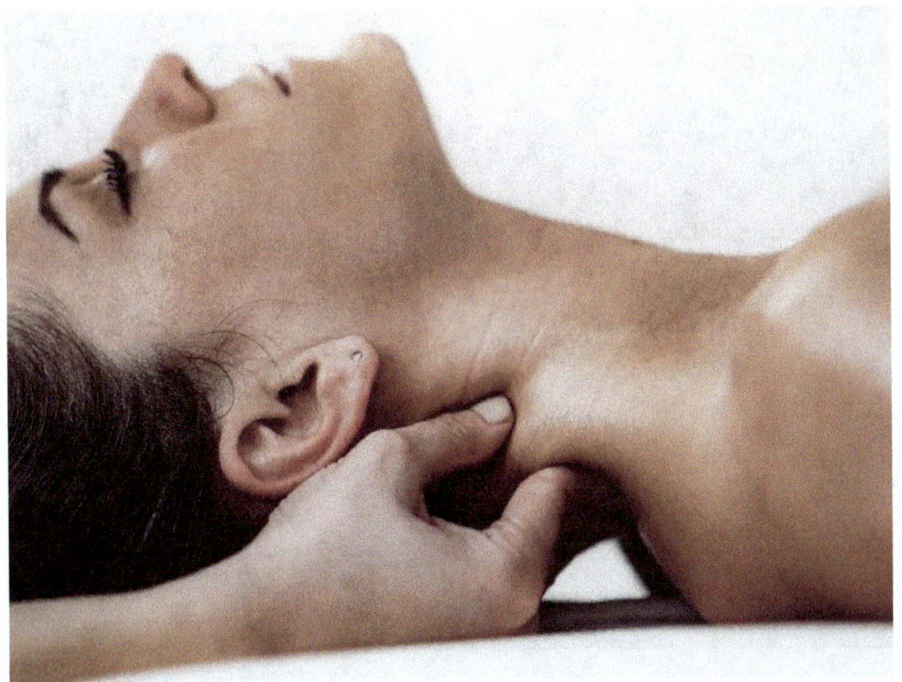

13. Abhyanga oil massage

Abhyanga is a type of oil massage from the system of Ayurvedic medicine. The oil is warmed and gently massaged all over the body. This type of massage focuses on nourishing the skin rather than deeply massaging the muscles. Benefits include:

- reduced stress

- activation of the parasympathetic nervous system (rest and digest)

- improved skin health and moisture

- reduced blood pressure

- reduced muscle stiffness

Abhyanga can be done by oneself or by a qualified practitioner. These massages usually last 60 minutes or longer.

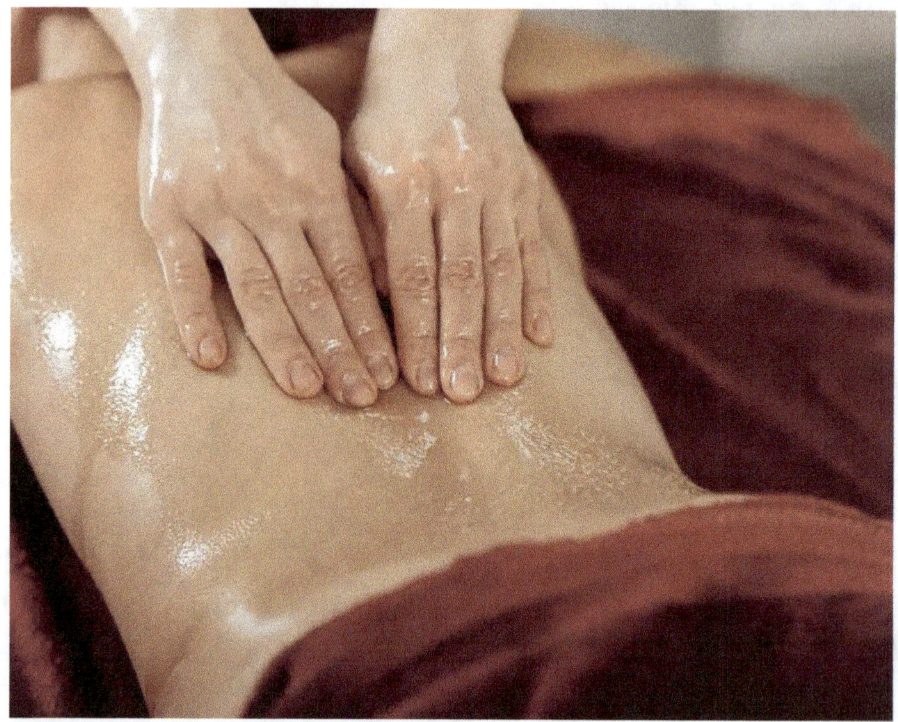

14. Myofascial release therapy

Myofascial release therapy is a type of bodywork that involves releasing stiffness in the fascia, the connective tissue system that contains each muscle in the body. Your therapist will massage and stretch any areas that feel tense with light pressure.

Specific conditions that may benefit from myofascial therapy include:

- myofascial pain syndrome

- headaches

- venous insufficiency

- If one experiences any of the following, cranial sacral therapy may not be for appropriate for them:

- severe bleeding disorders

- a diagnosed aneurysm

- a history of recent traumatic head injuries, which may include cranial bleeding or skull fractures

These massages usually last 60 minutes or longer.

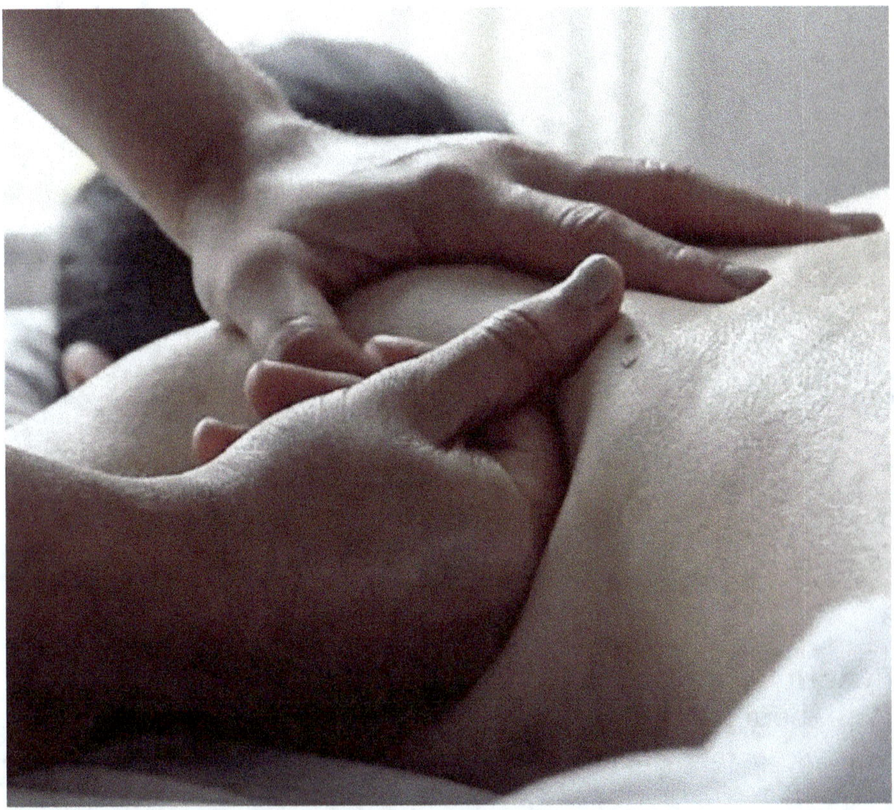

15. Craniosacral Therapy

Craniosacral therapy is a gentle, non-invasive way to release stress in the craniosacral system, which comprises the bones, tissues, and fluid surrounding the brain and spinal cord. Through light touch and manipulation, this treatment improves the body's ability to heal, helps people relax deeply, and brings them back into balance. This practice is mostly used to treat headaches, migraines, neck and back pain, stress-related disorders, temporomandibular joint (TMJ) dysfunction, and certain neurological conditions. During a cranial sacral massage session, a trained therapist uses light touch and subtle movements to assess and address any imbalances or restrictions in the craniosacral system. The craniosacral system includes the membranes and cerebrospinal fluid that surround and protect the brain and spinal cord.

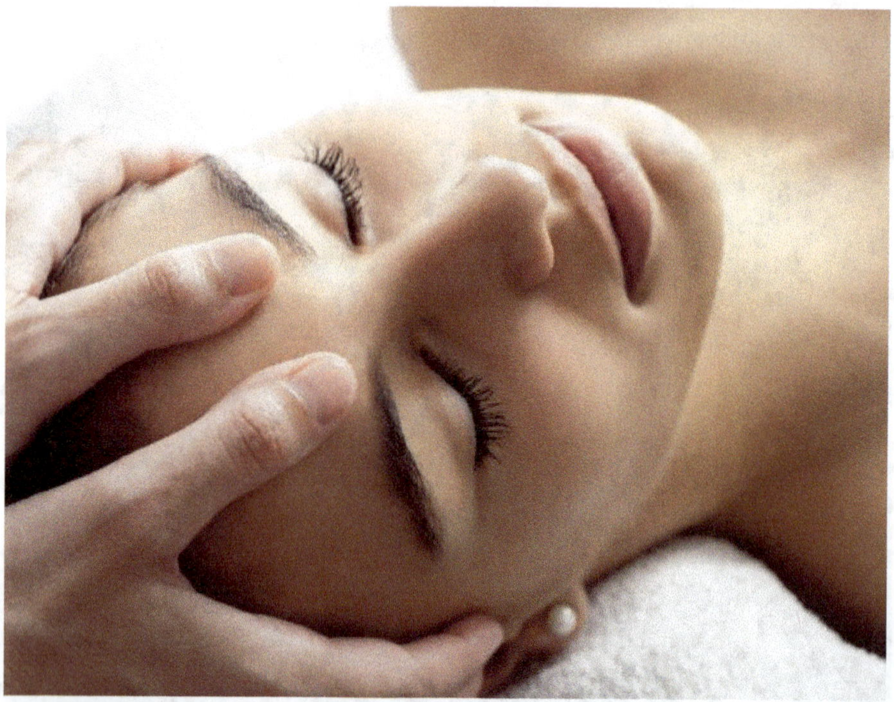

Benefits of Massage for Physical, Emotional, and Mental Well-being

Massage therapy offers a wealth of benefits for both the body and mind. From relieving muscle tension to enhancing mood and promoting relaxation, massage is a powerful tool for overall well-being.

Physical Benefits:

- **Pain Relief:** One of the most immediate and noticeable benefits of massage is pain relief. Whether you're dealing with chronic back pain, tension headaches, or muscle soreness, massage can target the source of the pain and help relieve it.

- **Improved Circulation:** Massage helps increase blood flow, which delivers oxygen and nutrients to the muscles and tissues.

This improved circulation can help speed up the healing process and enhance overall physical health.

- **Increased Flexibility and Range of Motion:** By loosening tight muscles and joints, massage helps improve flexibility and range of motion. This is particularly beneficial for athletes or individuals with stiffness or limited mobility.

- **Boosted Immune System:** Regular massage has been shown to enhance immune function by increasing lymph flow, which helps the body fight off infections and illnesses more effectively.

- **Reduced Muscle Tension and Stress:** Massage can help relieve chronic tension in muscles, reducing stiffness and discomfort. It also helps release lactic acid and toxins that build up in the muscles during physical activity.

Emotional and Mental Benefits:

- **Stress Reduction:** Massage is widely known for its ability to reduce stress levels by lowering cortisol, the body's primary stress hormone. Regular massage sessions help the body enter a state of deep relaxation, counteracting the effects of stress and promoting a sense of calm.

- **Improved Mood:** By triggering the release of endorphins (the body's natural "feel-good" chemicals), massage can improve mood and decrease feelings of anxiety or depression. This emotional lift is one of the reasons why massage therapy is used as a treatment for mental health issues.

- **Better Sleep:** Many people find that massage improves the quality of their sleep. By relaxing the body and mind, massage helps reduce insomnia and other sleep disturbances, making it easier to fall asleep and stay asleep.

- **Enhanced Mindfulness and Awareness:** Massage can encourage mindfulness by helping individuals become more aware of their bodies, their tension, and their emotional state. This awareness promotes relaxation and can help people release pent-up emotions.

- **Emotional Release:** Deep tissue and trigger point massage techniques can often release not only physical tension but also emotional tension. Sometimes, individuals may experience emotional responses during or after a session, as the body releases stress that has been stored in muscles.

Conclusion: A Healing Touch for Body and Mind

Massage therapy is much more than a luxurious treat or a way to pass the time—it's a powerful tool for enhancing overall health and well-being. By understanding the core principles behind massage, the different types of techniques available, and the wide-ranging benefits, you can begin to appreciate the value of this ancient healing art.

Whether you're seeking relief from physical pain, emotional stress, or mental fatigue, massage therapy offers a holistic approach to healing that nurtures the body, mind, and spirit. It's not just about physical touch; it's about the profound connection between therapist and client, a connection that has the power to restore balance and bring peace.

As you continue your exploration of massage, remember that the healing process is as much about the journey as it is about the destination. Each touch, each stroke, and each session brings you closer to understanding the full potential of this transformative practice.

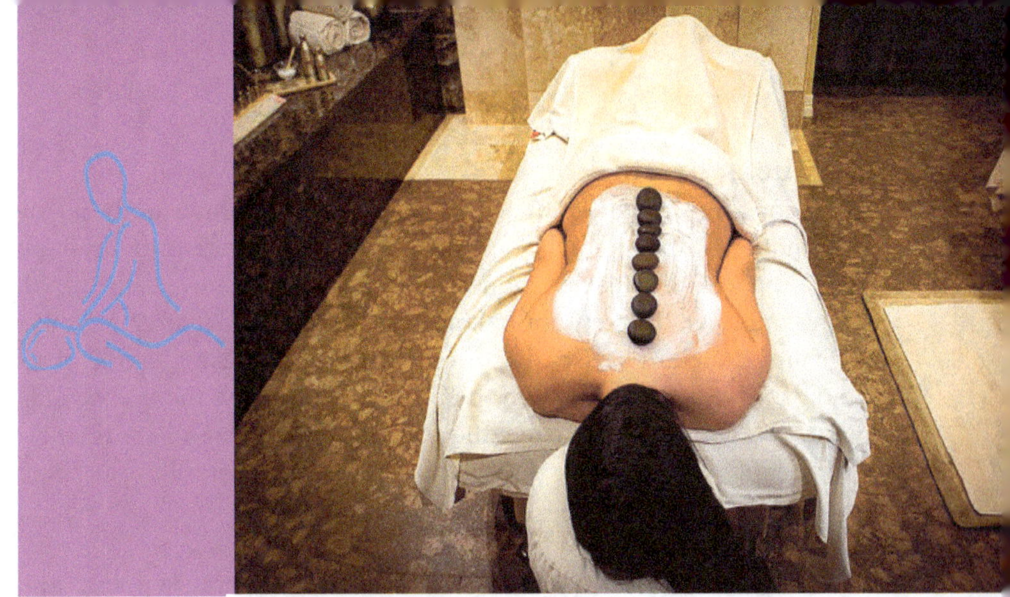

2

ANATOMY BASICS FOR MASSAGE PRACTITIONERS

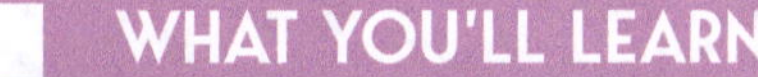

WHAT YOU'LL LEARN

◊ KEY MUSCLE GROUPS AND THEIR FUNCTONS

◊ UNDERSTANDING PRESSURE POINTS AND

ENERGY PATHWAYS

◊ HOW MASSAGE IMPACTS CIRCULATION,

LYMPHATIC DRAINAGE & NERVOUS SYSTEM

FUNCTION

Know the Body, Heal the Body

As a massage practitioner, understanding the human body is the foundation upon which you build your skill set. The body is an intricate system of muscles, bones, nerves, and energy pathways, all working together to maintain balance and function. To offer effective and healing touch, it's essential to recognize how these systems work and how massage interacts with them. When you know the body inside and out, you can apply your techniques with precision and confidence, knowing that you are aiding the healing process and helping your client restore balance.

In this chapter, we will explore key muscle groups, pressure points, and energy pathways within the body, giving you a deeper understanding of how to target areas for healing. We will also dive into the physical effects of massage on the body, including its impact on circulation, lymphatic drainage, and the nervous system. Whether you are a seasoned practitioner or just starting out, having this knowledge will enhance your massage practice and make it more effective for those you treat.

Key Muscle Groups and Their Functions

Understanding the major muscle groups in the body is crucial for delivering a massage that effectively targets tension and promotes healing. Muscles are responsible for movement, stability, and maintaining posture, and when they become tight or overworked, they can lead to pain and dysfunction. Let's look at some of the key muscle groups and their functions:

1. Neck and Shoulders:

The neck and shoulder muscles are some of the most commonly affected by stress and tension. These muscles often become tight due to poor posture, prolonged sitting, or emotional stress. The key muscles in this area include:

- **Trapezius:** This large muscle spans the upper back and neck, playing a crucial role in moving and stabilizing the shoulder blades and neck. It is commonly affected by stress and tension, leading to stiff necks or shoulder pain.

- **Levator Scapulae:** This muscle runs from the cervical spine to the shoulder blade and helps lift the shoulder. It often tightens up from poor posture or repetitive movements.

- **Sternocleidomastoid:** This muscle runs along the sides of the neck and is involved in rotating and tilting the head. It is often affected by tension, especially when people spend long hours looking at screens or sitting in one position.

Massage techniques targeting these muscles help relieve stiffness, promote relaxation, and improve the range of motion in the neck and shoulders. Applying slow, deliberate pressure can also help to reduce headaches that stem from muscle tension in this region.

2. Back Muscles:

The back is home to many important muscle groups that provide stability and allow for movement. Some of the key muscles in the back include:

- **Latissimus Dorsi:** These large, flat muscles cover much of the lower back and are responsible for shoulder and arm movements. Tightness here can lead to back pain or discomfort during daily activities.

- **Rhomboids:** Located between the shoulder blades, the rhomboids are important for retracting the shoulder blades and maintaining good posture. They are often tight in individuals who sit for long periods or perform repetitive tasks.

- **Erector Spinae:** Running along the length of the spine, the erector spinae muscles are responsible for keeping the spine erect and allowing for bending and twisting movements. They are key muscles to address when working with back pain or stiffness.

Massage on the back helps alleviate tension in these muscles, improve flexibility, and promote better posture. Techniques such as kneading and friction can reach deep into these muscle groups, providing effective relief.

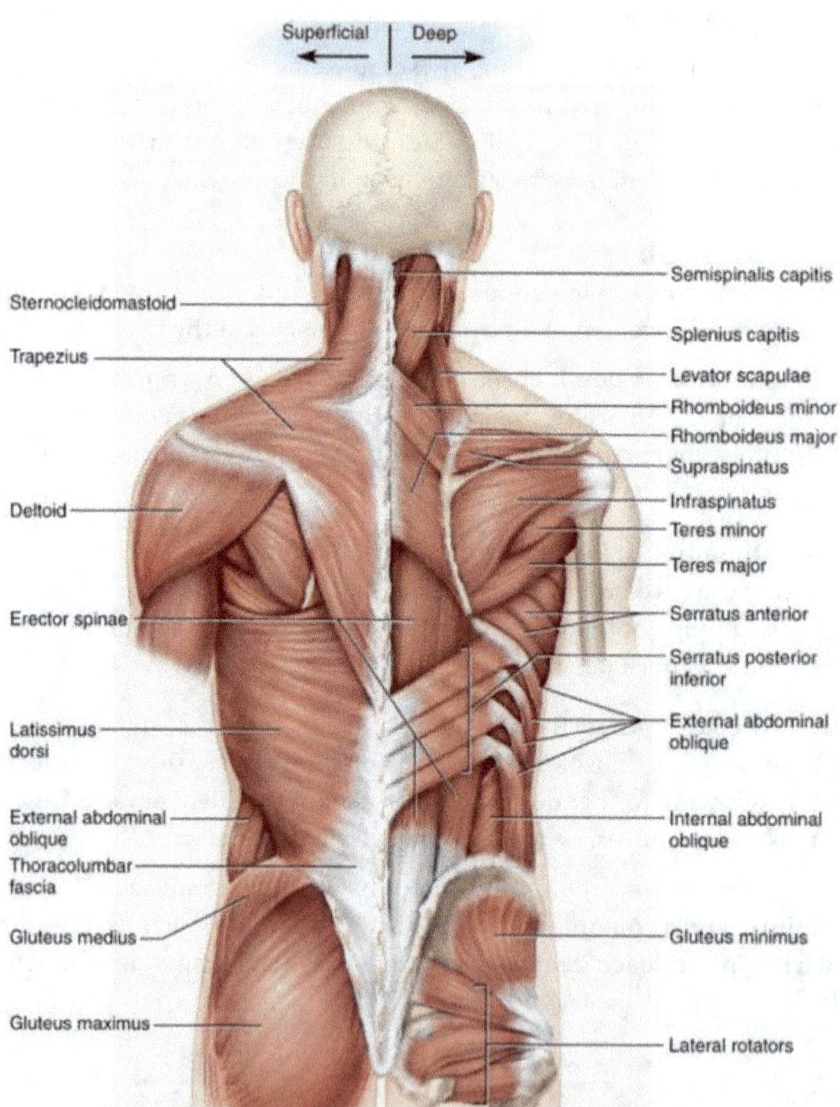

Superficial | Deep
Semispinalis capitis
Sternocleidomastoid
Splenius capitis
Trapezius
Levator scapulae
Rhomboideus minor
Rhomboideus major
Supraspinatus
Infraspinatus
Deltoid
Teres minor
Teres major
Erector spinae
Serratus anterior
Serratus posterior inferior
External abdominal oblique
Latissimus dorsi
External abdominal oblique
Internal abdominal oblique
Thoracolumbar fascia
Gluteus medius
Gluteus minimus
Gluteus maximus
Lateral rotators

3. Lower Body:

The muscles of the lower body are crucial for mobility and movement. Some of the most important muscles in the legs and lower body include:

- **Gluteus Maximus:** This large muscle forms the bulk of the buttocks and is essential for hip extension, standing up, and walking. Tightness in the glutes can lead to lower back pain and discomfort while sitting.

- **Hamstrings:** Located at the back of the thighs, the hamstrings play a key role in bending the knee and extending the hip. They are often tight with individuals who sit for long periods or engage in activities like running or cycling.

- **Quadriceps:** The quadriceps are the large muscles on the front of the thigh and are responsible for extending the knee. They are often tight in athletes or those who engage in repetitive leg movements.

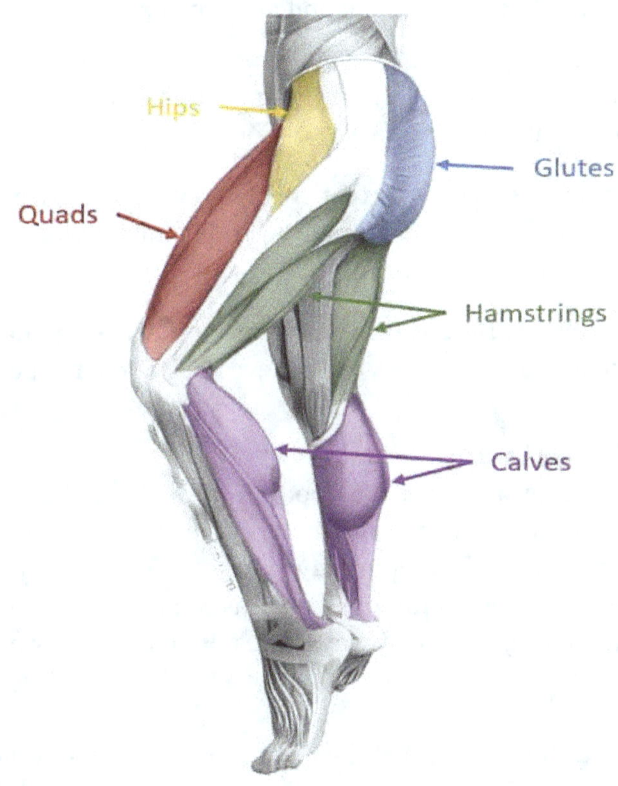

Focusing on these muscles during a massage session can relieve tension, enhance mobility, and promote circulation. Stretching and kneading techniques are especially effective in releasing tightness in the legs and glutes.

Understanding Pressure Points and Energy Pathways

In addition to knowing the muscles, it's essential to understand the concept of pressure points and energy pathways in the body. These concepts are particularly important when performing techniques like acupressure or shiatsu, where the practitioner applies pressure to specific points along the body to promote healing.

1. Pressure Points:

Pressure points are specific spots on the body that are known to be sensitive to touch. These points are often located along muscle groups, tendons, and ligaments, and they correspond to various areas of tension or discomfort. By applying targeted pressure to these points, a massage therapist can release built-up tension and alleviate pain.

For example:

- **The base of the skull** is a common pressure point for relieving headaches or neck pain.

- **The palms and soles of the feet** contain several pressure points that correspond to different parts of the body and are often used in reflexology to improve overall health.

- **The trapezius muscle** at the top of the shoulders often harbors tight spots that, when targeted, can relieve neck and back pain.

2. Energy Pathways (Meridians):

In traditional Chinese medicine, the body is thought to have energy pathways, or meridians, through which life energy (or Qi) flows. Blockages or imbalances in this energy flow can lead to physical or emotional issues. Massage techniques, such as Shiatsu or acupressure, are based on stimulating these pathways to restore balance and promote healing.

For example, the **Gallbladder Meridian** runs along the sides of the body and affects areas like the shoulders, neck, and hips. When blocked, it can contribute to stiffness and pain. By applying pressure along these meridians, massage practitioners can restore the flow of energy, alleviate tension, and improve overall health.

While the concept of energy pathways may seem abstract, it has been practiced for centuries and has proven to be an effective method of healing. Understanding these pathways allows you to take a more holistic approach to your massage practice.

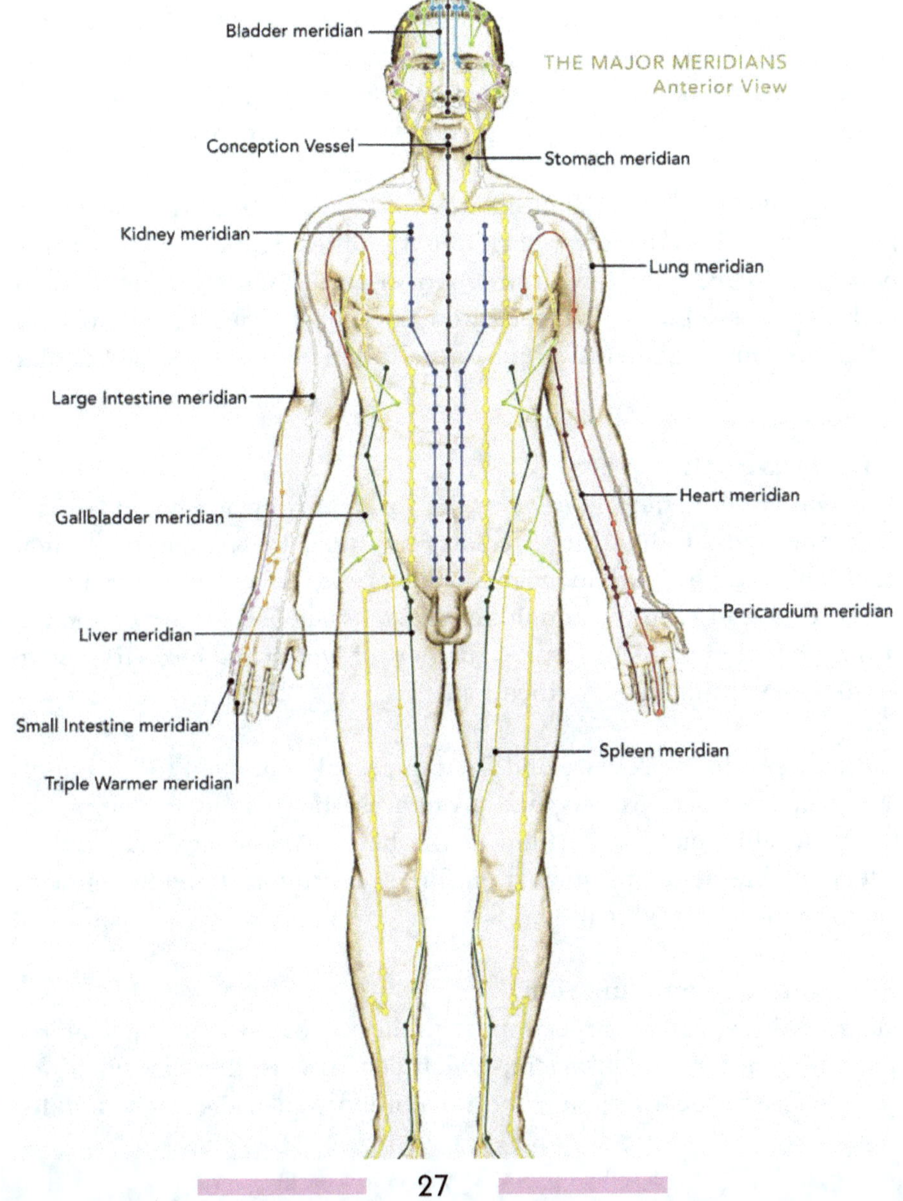

How Massage Impacts Circulation, Lymphatic Drainage and Nervous System Function

Massage therapy goes beyond just releasing muscle tension—it has a profound impact on the body's internal systems. The benefits of massage reach deep into the circulatory, lymphatic, and nervous systems, promoting health and well-being.

1. Circulation:

One of the primary benefits of massage is the stimulation of circulation. When pressure is applied to the muscles during massage, blood flow is temporarily increased to that area. This increase in blood circulation helps to deliver oxygen and nutrients to the tissues and removes waste products, which is especially important for muscle recovery.

Massage also improves the circulation of blood in areas that may have poor flow, such as the lower back or extremities. This can be especially beneficial for individuals with circulatory issues, such as poor circulation in the legs or swelling in the feet. By encouraging the heart to pump more efficiently, massage helps optimize the function of the cardiovascular system.

2. Lymphatic Drainage:

The lymphatic system is responsible for removing toxins and waste from the body. Unlike the circulatory system, the lymphatic system does not have a pump (like the heart), so it relies on movement and body compression to keep the lymph flowing. Massage, especially lymphatic drainage techniques, encourages the flow of lymph and helps to reduce swelling and promote detoxification.

For example, light pressure and rhythmic strokes applied to the lymph nodes in the neck, armpits, and groin areas help stimulate lymphatic flow and eliminate excess fluid in the body. This makes massage an effective treatment for reducing puffiness, improving immune function, and promoting detoxification.

3. Nervous System Function:

Massage therapy has a direct impact on the nervous system, particularly the autonomic nervous system, which controls involuntary functions such as heart rate, digestion, and respiration. When the body is under stress, the sympathetic nervous system (the "fight or flight" response) becomes activated, leading to heightened stress and tension. Massage activates the parasympathetic nervous system, which promotes relaxation and the "rest and digest" response.

This shift from sympathetic to parasympathetic activation helps to lower heart rate, reduce blood pressure, and promote overall relaxation. Additionally, massage can help with conditions related to nervous system dysfunction, such as anxiety, insomnia, and muscle spasms. Techniques like slow, rhythmic strokes and deep tissue work help to calm the nervous system and restore balance to the body.

Conclusion

Anatomy knowledge is the backbone of any effective massage practice. By understanding key muscle groups, pressure points, and energy pathways, you can target the right areas of the body to promote healing, alleviate pain, and improve overall well-being. Additionally, understanding how massage affects the circulatory, lymphatic, and nervous systems allows you to take a more holistic approach to your treatments. With this knowledge, you will not only be able to perform better massages, but you will also deepen your connection to the healing power of touch.

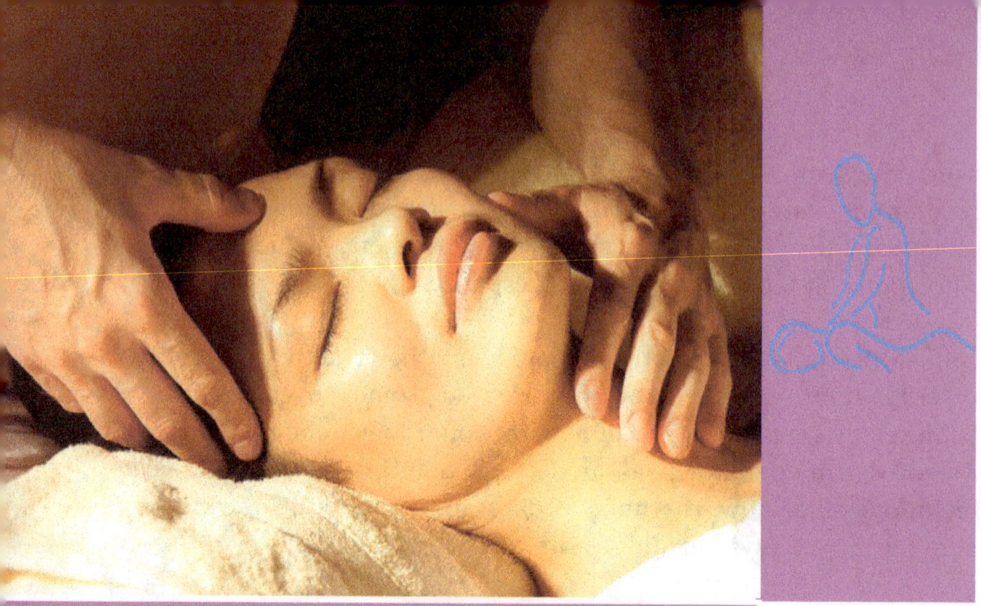

3

CORE MASSAGE TECHNIQUES

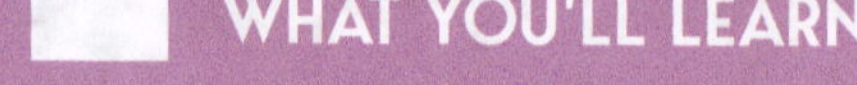

WHAT YOU'LL LEARN

◊ THE FIVE CORE MASSAGE STROKES

◊ TECHNQUES FOR APPLYING APPROPRIATE

PRESSURE AND RHYTHM

◊ ADAPTING TECHNIQUES FOR DIFFERENT BODY

TYPES AND PREFERENCES

Building Blocks of Effective Massage

In this Chapter we'll dive into the essential techniques that form the backbone of any good massage. Whether you're looking to enhance your skills for personal use or professional practice, understanding the core strokes and movements is the key to providing effective and soothing massages.

Massage isn't just about relaxing; it's a powerful tool for improving well-being, easing muscle tension, reducing stress, and even improving circulation. The movements you use in a massage work together to encourage healing, release tightness, and restore balance. This chapter is all about building the right foundation, helping you develop confidence in your technique, and ensuring you're applying the right pressure and rhythm for the best results.

Let's explore the five core massage strokes that are the heart of effective massage. We'll cover each stroke in depth, discuss when and why to use them, and how to adjust your approach to different needs and body types.

1. Effleurage: The Gentle Glide

Effleurage is the French word for "gliding" and is one of the most common strokes used in massage. It's often the first technique you'll use when starting a session, and it serves a few key purposes: it warms up the muscles, introduces the client to your touch, and helps to prepare the body for deeper work.

What it is:

Effleurage is a long, smooth, and gentle gliding stroke that covers large areas of the body, such as the back, legs, or arms. You use the palms of your hands or the pads of your fingers to glide smoothly along the skin, creating a soft and soothing rhythm.

How to apply it:

To perform effleurage, use light to moderate pressure as you move your hands in long, flowing strokes. Start from one area (like the lower back or the calves) and glide up toward the heart, following the natural flow of blood circulation. This helps to stimulate blood flow and relaxes the nervous system.

Effleurage isn't just a prelude to other techniques; it can also be used throughout the massage to reintroduce calm or to "reset" the body between more intense movements. It's gentle and relaxing, perfect for reducing stress or for those new to massage.

When to use it:
Effleurage is best used at the beginning and end of a session to relax the body and set the tone. It can also be used as a transitional stroke between deeper techniques, giving the client a moment to relax before you continue with the session.

2. Petrissage: The Kneading and Lifting Technique

Petrissage (pronounced pet-rih-sahzh) is another classic massage stroke that involves kneading and lifting the muscles. It's a more intensive technique compared to effleurage and is especially useful for working out tension and improving muscle tone.

What it is:
Petrissage involves kneading, rolling, and lifting the soft tissues of the body. It's like giving your muscles a gentle but firm squeeze, working to release tightness and break down knots. This technique targets the deeper layers of muscle tissue, making it ideal for areas of chronic tension, such as the shoulders, neck, or thighs.

How to apply it:
To perform petrissage, you can use the heels of your hands, your thumbs, or your fingers to knead the muscles. Think of it like kneading dough: apply pressure, lift and roll the tissue, and release. The rhythm can vary—sometimes you'll use deep pressure, while other times, a lighter touch may be more appropriate, depending on the client's needs.

When to use it:
Petrissage is particularly useful for working out muscle knots or areas that feel tight. It's great for larger muscle groups like the thighs, calves, or upper back. However, because it's more intense, you'll want to use this technique with care, ensuring that the client is comfortable and that you're not applying too much pressure on more delicate areas.

3. Friction: The Therapeutic Rubbing Technique

Friction is a massage technique designed to reach deep into the muscles and soft tissues. It's often used to target specific knots or adhesions that can form in the muscles or connective tissue.

What it is:

Friction involves small, deep, circular or back-and-forth movements with the fingers, palms, or thumbs. This technique doesn't involve sliding the hands over the body like effleurage, but instead focuses on applying direct pressure in small areas to release tension, adhesions, or tight spots.

How to apply it:

When performing friction, focus on the muscle fibers or specific areas of tension. Use your fingers or thumbs to apply deep pressure in small, circular motions or in short, back-and-forth strokes. The key is to apply enough pressure to work deeply into the tissue but not cause pain. It's a fine balance between effective pressure and comfort.

When to use it:

Friction is particularly helpful for working on chronic muscle pain, tension, or scar tissue. If you're working on someone with a knot or a muscle that's feeling particularly tight, friction can break down the tension and encourage the release of those stubborn areas. Use it sparingly, though, as it's a more intense technique.

4. Tapotement: The Rhythmic Tapping Technique

Tapotement is a fast, rhythmic technique that involves percussive movements. It's often used to stimulate the muscles and is great for invigorating the body, particularly after a deep tissue session.

What it is:

Tapotement involves quick, repeated tapping, chopping, or drumming motions with your hands. There are several variations of tapotement, including light tapping, hacking (like a karate chop), or cupping (where your hands form a cupping shape and tap lightly on the skin). This technique is energizing and promotes circulation, helping to "wake up" the muscles after deeper work.

How to apply it:
Use the edge of your hands, fingers, or the base of your palms to tap or drum rhythmically on the skin. The pressure is usually light but quick. You can adjust the speed depending on your client's comfort level and the areas you're focusing on. Tapotement is great for invigorating tired muscles or stimulating circulation in areas that need a little extra energy.

When to use it:
Tapotement is ideal toward the end of a session to "wake up" the body or to add some variety. It's great for refreshing the muscles, particularly the back, legs, or arms. However, you'll want to be mindful of the pressure you use—too hard, and it might cause discomfort; too soft, and it may not have the desired energizing effect.

5. Vibration: The Shaking and Relaxing Technique

Vibration involves gentle, rhythmic shaking or oscillation of the body or muscle groups. This technique is deeply soothing and can be incredibly effective in calming the nervous system and promoting relaxation.

What it is:
Vibration is a gentle shaking or oscillating motion applied to the muscles, either with your hands or through your whole body. The movement is soothing and helps release tension in a very calming way. It's particularly helpful in areas where the muscles are tight but sensitive to deep pressure.

How to apply it:
To perform vibration, use your palms or fingers to gently shake the body. You can do this by placing your hands on the muscles and gently applying a rocking motion or a slight oscillation. It's not about force; it's about providing a soothing, rhythmic movement that helps the body release tightness and relax deeply.

When to use it:
Vibration is often used at the end of a massage or when transitioning between different strokes. It's perfect for soothing the muscles after more intense work like deep tissue techniques. It also works well for clients who may be particularly sensitive or who need extra care in certain areas.

Techniques for Applying Appropriate Pressure and Rhythm

The effectiveness of a massage depends not only on the techniques used but also on how you apply them. Pressure and rhythm are crucial for delivering a massage that is both therapeutic and comfortable.

Pressure:

The amount of pressure you use depends on several factors, including the client's preferences, their body type, and the area being worked on. In general, you want to start light and progressively apply more pressure as the body relaxes. Use feedback from your client to gauge how much pressure they are comfortable with. Some areas of the body, like the back and thighs, may handle more pressure, while others, like the neck or abdomen, may need a lighter touch.

Rhythm:

Rhythm is just as important as pressure. A steady, consistent rhythm helps to calm the nervous system, while abrupt changes in speed can create discomfort or tension. As you perform your strokes, maintain a smooth and flowing rhythm, whether you're doing the gentle glide of effleurage or the deeper kneading of petrissage. A steady rhythm helps the client relax and trust the process, leading to a more enjoyable experience.

Adapting Techniques for Different Body Types and Preferences

Every person is unique, and understanding how to adapt your techniques for different body types and preferences is essential for an effective massage.

Body Types:

Not all bodies respond to massage in the same way. For example, someone with a lot of muscle mass might need firmer pressure to feel the benefits, while someone with less muscle tone might prefer a gentler touch. Adjust your pressure and technique to suit the individual. When working with larger body types, you may need to apply more pressure for effective results, while on smaller body types, lighter strokes can be more appropriate.

Personal Preferences:
Some clients may have specific preferences about how they like their massages. Whether they prefer lighter strokes, deeper pressure, or a specific focus on certain areas, always take the time to check in with them. Ask about any areas that need special attention, or whether there are areas to avoid.

Conclusion

Mastering these core techniques will help you build a solid foundation for any massage practice, whether for yourself or others. Each of these strokes—effleurage, petrissage, friction, tapotement, and vibration—can be used to target different needs and provide various benefits. Remember, the key to effective massage is not only in the strokes you use but also in how you apply pressure, maintain rhythm, and adapt your approach to the individual you're working with.

With these techniques in your toolbox, you're well on your way to becoming a confident, skilled practitioner. Now, let's move forward and start putting it all into practice.

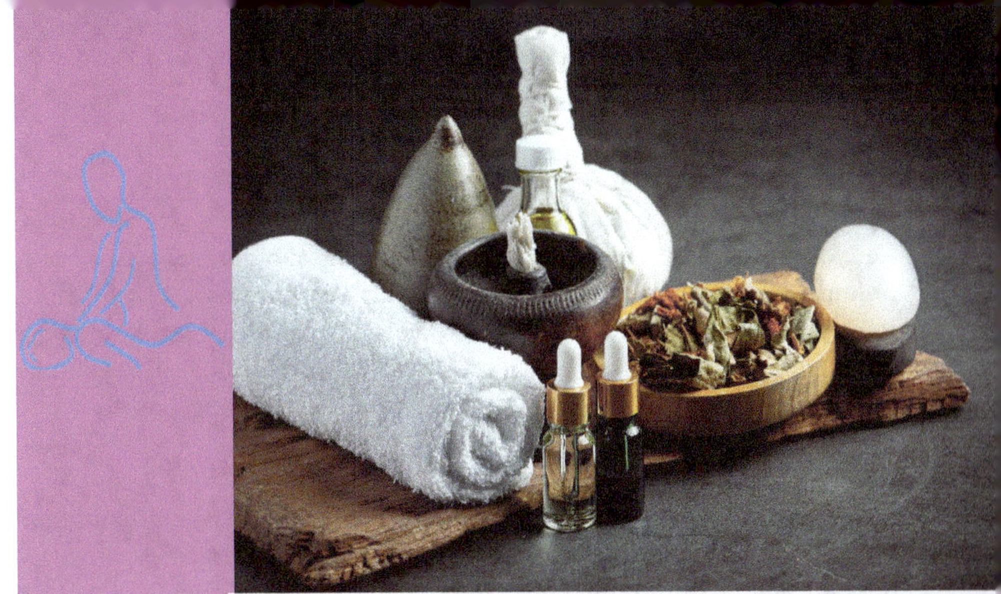

4

TOOLS, MATERIALS AND ENVIRONMENT

WHAT YOU'LL LEARN

◊ CHOOSNG THE RIGHT OILS, CREAMS AND TOOLS

◊ PREPARING YOUR SPACE

◊ HYGIENE AND PROFESSIONALISM

Equipping Yourself for Success

This chapter focuses on the tools and environment that can elevate your practice. The right tools, materials, and a peaceful, well-organized environment will ensure that you create a comfortable, therapeutic experience for yourself or your clients. When every element of your massage setup is considered and prepared with care, you can achieve more effective results and create a calming, professional experience that everyone will enjoy.

Let's explore the essential elements: choosing the right oils, creams, and tools; preparing your space to make it as soothing and functional as possible; and maintaining high standards of hygiene and professionalism to keep your practice safe and successful.

Choosing the Right Oils, Creams and Tools

When it comes to massage, oils and creams are more than just a luxury—they're a necessity. The right choice will ensure that your strokes flow smoothly, provide proper hydration to the skin, and enhance the overall massage experience. But with so many options available, how do you know which ones to choose? Here's what you need to know.

Oils and Creams:

Massage oils and creams help reduce friction and allow your hands to glide smoothly across the skin. They also nourish and hydrate the skin, which can be especially beneficial for dry skin or during longer sessions. Here are some of the most common types:

- **Carrier Oils:** These are the base oils, like coconut oil, almond oil, jojoba oil, and grapeseed oil. Each has its own properties, such as hydration, soothing effects, or anti-inflammatory benefits. For example, coconut oil is often favored for its natural antibacterial properties, while jojoba oil is great for skin hydration without feeling too greasy.

- **Essential Oils:** These oils are highly concentrated extracts from plants that provide specific therapeutic benefits, such as lavender for relaxation, peppermint for muscle relief, or eucalyptus for clearing respiratory passages. When using essential oils, always dilute them with a carrier oil to avoid skin irritation.

- **Creams and Lotions:** If you're working with someone who doesn't like the feel of oil or prefers a lighter texture, you might want to consider massage creams or lotions. These often absorb more quickly than oils, leaving less residue, and they can provide a smoother, more comfortable glide, especially in cooler environments.

Tools:

While oils and creams are vital, there are a few additional tools that can enhance your technique and bring extra benefits to the table. Here are a few commonly used massage tools:

- **Massage Stones:** Heated stones can provide soothing warmth to tense muscles, while cold stones can be used for reducing inflammation or increasing circulation. Hot stone massages are particularly relaxing and offer a deep, penetrating warmth.

- **Massage Balls or Rollers:** These tools are great for self-massage or for applying deep pressure to smaller, specific areas like the shoulders or feet. They can also be used as an alternative to your hands when working on tough knots or tight spots.

- **Massage Tables and Chairs:** If you're working professionally, a sturdy, adjustable massage table is key for comfort, both for you and your client. If you're working on a smaller scale, like with a partner or at home, portable massage chairs or cushions can be great alternatives.

When to Choose Each Tool:

Ultimately, the choice between oils, creams, or tools comes down to your goals for the massage, the preferences of the person you're massaging, and the area being worked on. Lighter oils work well for gentle strokes, while heavier oils or creams may be better for deeper tissue work. Similarly, tools like massage balls and stones are excellent for targeting specific tension areas, offering deeper pressure, or enhancing the overall experience.

Preparing Your Space: Creating a Relaxing and Functional Environment

The environment you create is just as important as the techniques and tools you use. The right setting can make a huge difference in how someone feels during and after a massage. Whether you're offering massage in a professional setting or just at home, creating a calming and functional space will help your recipient relax and get the most out of the experience.

A Calm, Inviting Atmosphere:

Start by ensuring the space is clean, clutter-free, and comfortable. This will allow both you and the person you're massaging to focus on the massage itself without distractions. Consider the following:

- **Lighting:** Soft, dim lighting helps create a relaxing atmosphere. Avoid bright overhead lights, and instead, opt for warm lamps, candles, or natural light, if possible. You can also use Himalayan salt lamps, which offer a calming glow.

- **Music:** Background music can help set the tone. Slow, instrumental music or nature sounds like ocean waves or birds chirping can soothe the mind and body. Make sure the volume is low and steady so it doesn't distract from the massage.

- **Aromatherapy:** If you're using essential oils, consider adding a diffuser to your space. Scents like lavender, chamomile, or sandalwood can calm the mind and promote relaxation. Just be mindful of sensitivities or allergies to certain scents.

- **Comfortable Setup:** If you're working on a massage table, make sure it's adjusted for comfort, with soft, clean linens. A towel or blanket can help provide warmth and ensure your client feels supported. If you're working with someone on the floor, make sure there are thick mats or cushions for a comfortable session.

Functional Setup:

While creating a serene atmosphere is important, the space should also be functional and organized. Ensure you have easy access to all the tools and products you need during the session. Here are a few practical tips:

- **Keep Massage Tools Nearby:** Make sure you have oils, towels, and any massage tools easily accessible to avoid interruptions during the massage. A small table next to the massage area can be handy for holding everything.

- **Space for Movement:** If you're working with a partner or client, there should be enough space for you to move around comfortably and adjust your position as needed. You should be able to access different areas of the body easily, from the shoulders to the legs, without feeling cramped or restricted.

- **Temperature Control:** Ensure that the room is comfortably warm. A cold environment can cause muscles to tighten, while a warm environment helps muscles relax. Use a space heater or blankets to maintain a cozy, comfortable temperature.

Hygiene and Professionalism for Effective and Safe Practice

Hygiene is a critical part of massage, not only for the comfort and safety of your clients or partners but also for your own well-being. Whether you're massaging professionally or just offering a therapeutic experience at home, maintaining cleanliness and professionalism will help ensure a positive experience.

Personal Hygiene:

Before beginning any massage, make sure your hands are clean and free of any lotions or oils you don't intend to use. Keep your nails trimmed and clean, and avoid wearing any jewelry that could dig into the skin during the massage. If you're massaging professionally, consider wearing clean, comfortable clothing or a uniform that allows freedom of movement.

Clean Environment:

After every session, make sure the massage table or area is cleaned and disinfected. If you're using oils, creams, or lotions, wipe down surfaces to avoid residue buildup. Clean towels should be used for each session, and anything that comes in contact with skin (such as sheets or massage tools) should be laundered regularly.

Disinfecting Tools:

Massage stones, balls, and other tools should be disinfected after each use, especially when working with clients. This is especially important for shared equipment, as it ensures that you maintain a hygienic environment for every session. A simple disinfecting solution will do the job, but be sure to follow the manufacturer's care instructions for each tool.

Maintaining Professional Boundaries:

Whether you're massaging friends, family, or clients, maintaining professionalism is key. Always establish clear communication and set expectations for the session. Make sure the client feels comfortable and is aware of the level of pressure being applied. It's also important to respect personal boundaries, ensuring that the massage experience remains relaxing and safe for everyone involved.

Conclusion

Creating the right environment and using the best tools and materials will elevate your massage practice, whether you're performing it on yourself, a loved one, or a client. The proper oils, lotions, and tools will not only improve your technique but also add to the overall experience. At the same time, a relaxing, functional environment and high standards of hygiene and professionalism will ensure that your practice remains effective, safe, and enjoyable for everyone involved.

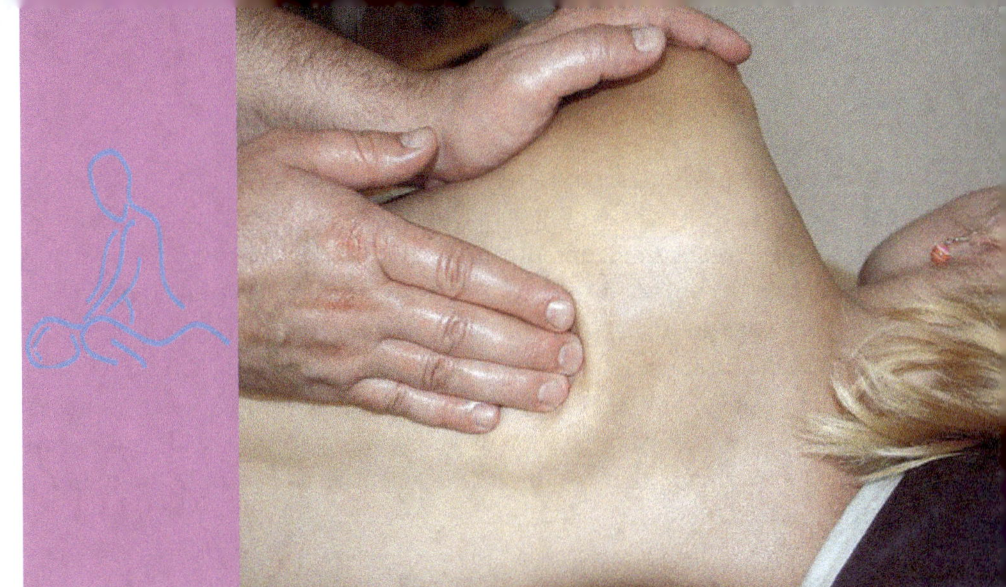

5

MASSAGE FOR STRESS MANAGEMENT

 **WHAT YOU'LL LEARN** 

◇ HOW TO RELEASE TENSION IN KEY AREAS

◇ INCORPRATING BREATHING TECHNIQUES

AND MINDFULNESS

◇ METHODS FOR CREATING A DEEPLY

RELAXING EXPERIENCE

Calming the Mind and Body

In this Chapter, we explore one of the most powerful benefits of massage: stress management. In today's fast-paced world, stress has become a major part of daily life, affecting our physical and mental well-being. But the good news is that massage is one of the most effective ways to alleviate stress and calm the mind and body. Whether you're giving a massage for relaxation or addressing specific areas of tension, the techniques we discuss here will help guide you in providing a deeply relaxing experience that can melt away stress and bring the body into a state of peace.

Stress manifests in different ways for everyone, but common trouble spots include the neck, shoulders, and back—areas where tension tends to accumulate throughout the day. By learning how to release stress from these key areas and incorporating additional relaxation techniques like breathing and mindfulness, you can significantly reduce tension and help the body and mind feel more balanced.

Let's dive into how you can use massage as a tool for stress management and relaxation.

How to Release Tension in Key Areas: Neck, Shoulders, and Back

Stress often shows up in our muscles as tightness and discomfort, especially in the neck, shoulders, and back. These areas are particularly prone to tension because they carry much of the emotional and physical load of daily life. Whether from sitting at a desk all day, hunching over a phone, or carrying the weight of responsibilities, the muscles in these areas can become tense and stiff. Here's how to relieve that built-up tension using massage.

Neck: The neck is a common area for stress-related tension, especially due to poor posture or long periods of looking down at screens. This area can become stiff and painful, often causing headaches and discomfort in the shoulders.
To release tension in the neck:

- **Use Effleurage:** Start with gentle, soothing gliding strokes (effleurage) to warm up the area. Apply light pressure with your fingers or palms along the sides of the neck and the base of the skull, moving downward toward the shoulders.

- **Petrissage:** Use kneading strokes (petrissage) to gently lift and squeeze the neck muscles, focusing on any tight spots. Be careful not to apply too much pressure—this area is sensitive.

- **Circular Friction:** Use your fingertips or thumbs to apply deep circular friction to any knots or tension in the muscles at the back of the neck. This will help break down adhesions and promote relaxation.

Shoulders: The shoulders tend to carry a lot of tension, especially from stress or repetitive movements. If you notice tightness in this area, massaging the shoulders can significantly improve comfort and reduce stress.

To relieve shoulder tension:

- **Effleurage and Petrissage:** Start with gentle gliding (effleurage) to relax the area, followed by kneading strokes (petrissage) to target specific knots. Use your fingers or thumbs to work deep into the trapezius muscle (the large muscle in the upper back and shoulders), which often holds stress.

- **Tapping (Tapotement):** Tap the shoulders gently with the edges of your hands or fingers to stimulate circulation and bring relief to tight muscles.

Back: The back can store a lot of emotional tension, particularly in the upper and lower regions. Whether from poor posture or physical strain, back tension can create discomfort that affects overall well-being.

To release tension in the back:

- **Effleurage:** Start with smooth, gliding strokes over the upper back to relax the muscles.

- **Petrissage:** Apply deeper kneading pressure to the back, focusing on areas that feel tight, such as the lower back or the shoulder blades. Use your palms, thumbs, or knuckles to work deeply into these areas.

- **Frictions for Targeted Relief:** Use friction techniques on specific knots or stiff areas in the upper and lower back. This is especially helpful for tightness between the shoulder blades or in the lower back.

By focusing on these three key areas, you can help reduce the physical effects of stress and promote a feeling of overall relaxation.

Incorporating Breathing Techniques and Mindfulness During Massage

One of the most effective ways to enhance the stress-relieving benefits of massage is to incorporate mindfulness and breathing techniques. Both of these elements help activate the body's parasympathetic nervous system, which is responsible for the "rest and digest" response—helping the body relax and release tension. Here's how you can incorporate these techniques into your massage practice:

- **Breathing Techniques:** Breathing is deeply intertwined with stress and relaxation. Shallow, rapid breathing often accompanies stress, while slow, deep breaths activate the relaxation response. Teaching your client to focus on their breathing can help reduce stress and enhance the benefits of massage.

- **Slow, Deep Breathing:** Encourage your client to take slow, deep breaths throughout the session. Instruct them to inhale deeply through the nose for a count of four, hold for a count of four, and exhale slowly through the mouth for a count of six. This will calm the nervous system and help release physical tension.

- **Syncing Breath with Movement:** When performing strokes, synchronize your client's breathing with your movements. For example, encourage them to inhale as you glide your hands upward during effleurage, and exhale as you apply pressure or work downward. This rhythm helps deepen relaxation.

- **Abdominal Breathing:** If your client is feeling particularly tense, encourage them to place one hand on their abdomen and the other on their chest. Instruct them to breathe deeply, expanding the belly as they inhale and relaxing it as they exhale. This can help release stress, particularly in the chest and diaphragm areas.

Mindfulness and Relaxation: Incorporating mindfulness into the massage session helps your client stay present in the moment, rather than allowing their mind to wander to stressful thoughts. Guide them to focus on how their body feels and the sensations they're experiencing.

- **Guided Relaxation:** As you work on different areas of the body, encourage your client to mentally scan their body and notice where they may still be holding tension. Suggest they release that tension with each breath, relaxing their muscles consciously.

- **Positive Visualization:** Encourage your client to imagine relaxing imagery, like walking on a beach or lying in a sunlit garden. This mental imagery can promote relaxation and enhance the massage experience.

By combining massage techniques with focused breathing and mindfulness, you create a more profound and therapeutic experience that targets both the body and the mind. These techniques help guide the client into a deeper state of relaxation, allowing them to let go of stress and embrace the healing benefits of the massage.

Methods for Creating a Deeply Relaxing Experience for Your Client or Partner

Now that you've learned how to release tension and incorporate breathing and mindfulness techniques, let's focus on how to create an overall deeply relaxing experience. A truly effective massage goes beyond just the physical touch—it's about creating an environment and a presence that helps your client or partner feel safe, comfortable, and completely relaxed.

Setting the Mood: As discussed in Chapter 3, the environment plays a huge role in creating relaxation. A calm, peaceful space with dim lighting, soothing music, and calming scents will instantly help your client feel at ease. Take the time to prepare the room in advance, ensuring that it's quiet, comfortable, and free from distractions.

Engage the Senses: You can further enhance relaxation by engaging the senses in a gentle, non-overwhelming way:

- **Aromatherapy:** Use essential oils like lavender, chamomile, or eucalyptus to calm the mind and promote relaxation. A diffuser can disperse the scent throughout the room, adding to the soothing ambiance.

- **Sound:** Soft, instrumental music or nature sounds (rain, ocean waves, etc.) create a calming auditory experience that helps the mind settle into a relaxed state.

- **Touch:** Ensure that the massage itself is gentle and respectful of the person's boundaries. Adjust your pressure, rhythm, and technique based on their comfort level. Soft, rhythmic strokes like effleurage can be especially relaxing, while gentle kneading (petrissage) can help release deeper tension.

Creating Emotional Safety: Sometimes, emotional tension can be as present as physical tension. Always ask your client about their preferences and make sure they feel heard and safe throughout the session. Acknowledging their needs—whether it's focusing on a specific area or adjusting the pressure—helps to create an emotional space where they can fully let go.

Conclusion

Massage is a wonderful tool for stress management, offering relief not just for the body but for the mind as well. By focusing on releasing tension in the neck, shoulders, and back, and incorporating techniques like deep breathing and mindfulness, you'll provide a deeply relaxing and therapeutic experience. The key to stress management through massage is to slow down, listen to the body, and create a space that encourages deep relaxation and healing.

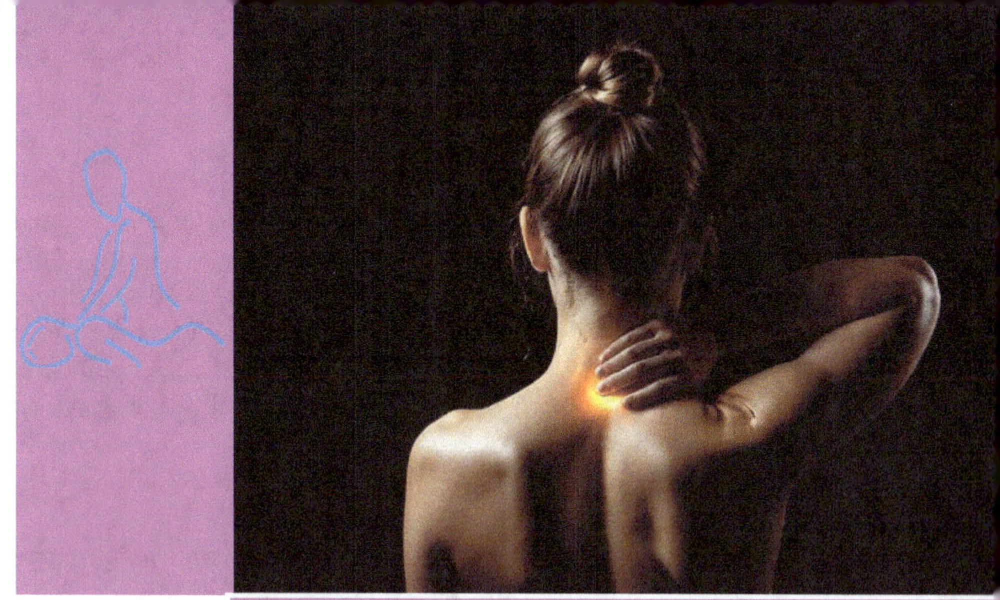

6

PAIN RELIEF AND REHABILITATION

WHAT YOU'LL LEARN

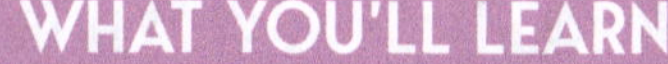

◊ TECHNIQUES FOR ADRESSING CHRONIC PAIN AND MUSCLE SORENESS

◊ SPECIALISED METHODS FOR FOR INJURIES, STIFFNESS AND JOINT PAIN

◊ WORKING WITH ATHLETES

Targeted Approaches for Healing

Now that you have an understanding of how massage can manage stress and promote relaxation, we're going to focus on one of its most powerful uses: **pain relief and rehabilitation.** Whether it's helping with chronic pain, muscle soreness, stiffness, or even recovering from an injury, massage therapy plays a critical role in reducing pain and aiding the body in its healing process. It is a tool that allows us to work directly with the body, using touch to promote better circulation, muscle function, and tissue repair.

Pain and discomfort are part of life, and many people experience different types of pain—from muscle soreness after exercise, to joint stiffness from long hours of sitting, to the more persistent, chronic pain of conditions like arthritis. No matter the source, massage can address the root causes and offer significant relief. In this chapter, we will explore a variety of techniques that are designed not only to alleviate pain but to help the body repair itself.

You will learn methods to ease chronic pain, address muscle soreness, aid in injury recovery, and provide relief from joint pain, all while working with individuals at different stages of healing. Additionally, you'll see how massage can help athletes before and after events, aiding in injury prevention and recovery. Let's dive into the ways massage can target and treat pain.

Techniques for Addressing Chronic Pain and Muscle Soreness

Chronic pain and muscle soreness are two of the most common reasons people seek out massage therapy. Chronic pain is often associated with long-term conditions like arthritis, fibromyalgia, or muscle imbalances, whereas muscle soreness typically results from physical activity, such as intense exercise, lifting, or prolonged sitting. Regardless of the cause, massage can be a highly effective remedy to ease discomfort and reduce tension.

Effleurage for Relaxation and Circulation:

Effleurage, which involves long, sweeping strokes, is one of the most basic massage techniques, and it's great for both relaxation and warming up the muscles. It helps stimulate blood flow to the area, which is essential for healing and reducing soreness. Effleurage can be performed lightly or with moderate pressure, depending on the condition of the muscles. For chronic pain or soreness, effleurage is typically used to begin the session, helping to loosen up the muscles before applying more intense techniques.

Start by using gentle strokes across the back, legs, arms, or neck, always in the direction of the heart to encourage circulation and lymphatic flow. This gentle approach helps increase warmth and prepares the muscles for deeper work.

Petrissage for Deeper Muscle Work:
Petrissage is the kneading technique that works deeply into the muscles, squeezing, lifting, and rolling the soft tissues. It's especially helpful for breaking down muscle knots and adhesions that contribute to pain and soreness. When muscles are in pain, the tissues become tight, and adhesions form, causing stiffness and discomfort. Petrissage helps to release these tight spots, improve flexibility, and restore natural muscle tone.

Focus on using both hands, or your fingers and thumbs, to gently knead the muscles. A deep kneading action works particularly well on larger muscle groups like the thighs, calves, and shoulders. You can alternate between gentle and firm pressure depending on the tolerance of your client.

Friction for Targeted Muscle Relief:
Friction involves applying concentrated, small, circular strokes to a specific area of muscle tension. This technique is ideal for breaking up adhesions or muscle knots that often accompany chronic pain. The key with friction is to apply firm pressure, using your fingertips or thumbs, and work in small circular or back-and-forth motions over the troubled area.

This method is great for focused pain relief in areas like the neck, upper back, and lower back, where tension tends to build up due to stress or poor posture. Friction helps stimulate blood flow to the muscles, which promotes healing and reduces discomfort. It's an ideal technique for those suffering from specific areas of tightness or muscle spasms.

Stretching for Flexibility:

Stretching is often an underutilized technique in traditional massage, but it plays an essential role in releasing muscle tension and increasing flexibility. When muscles become tight due to overuse or inactivity, they shorten, causing discomfort. Stretching during massage helps to lengthen the muscle, increase blood flow, and improve flexibility.

You can incorporate passive stretches into your massage routine by gently moving the client's limbs or torso in specific ways. For example, to stretch the hamstrings, you can lift the client's leg while they lie on their back, applying a gentle stretch to the back of their thigh. Stretching combined with massage encourages a faster recovery process, especially for athletes or people with chronic muscle tension.

Specialized Methods for Injuries, Stiffness and Joint Pain

In addition to addressing general soreness and chronic pain, massage can also be highly effective for those suffering from injuries, joint pain, or muscle stiffness. These conditions require specialized techniques to target the underlying causes and speed up recovery. Whether it's a muscle strain, joint stiffness from arthritis, or post-surgery rehabilitation, massage therapy can provide significant benefits.

Myofascial Release for Deep Tissue and Fascia:

Myofascial release is a specialized technique that focuses on the fascia—the connective tissue that surrounds muscles, bones, and organs. Often, after an injury or long-term muscle tension, the fascia becomes tight and restrictive, causing pain, stiffness, and limited mobility. By applying slow, sustained pressure to the fascia, myofascial release helps break up these adhesions, increasing flexibility and reducing pain.

This technique can be applied to specific areas of restriction, such as the lower back, hips, and shoulders. It's a gentle, yet deep technique that targets both the muscles and the fascia, allowing the body to relax and heal more effectively. It's particularly helpful for those recovering from injuries or surgeries where scar tissue and adhesions may have developed.

Joint Mobilization for Stiffness and Pain Relief:

Joint pain is a common concern, especially for people with arthritis or those recovering from an injury. Joint mobilization refers to the gentle, rhythmic movements of a joint to help improve its range of motion and reduce pain. For example, if your client has stiffness in their shoulder or knee, you can gently move the joint in its natural range of motion, applying light pressure to loosen up the joint and encourage fluid movement.

By improving joint mobility, you reduce the friction that causes pain and stiffness. Joint mobilization is a great technique for those with chronic conditions like arthritis, where inflammation and stiffness make it difficult to move freely.

Trigger Point Therapy for Pain Relief:
Trigger points are areas of muscle tissue that become tight and form "knots," which can refer pain to other areas of the body. For example, a tight spot in the neck may cause headaches, or a knot in the back may radiate pain into the hips. Trigger point therapy involves applying concentrated pressure directly on these points to release the muscle tension and alleviate pain.

To apply this technique, locate the trigger point by feeling for small, hard nodules in the muscle. Apply firm pressure directly on the spot, holding for 10–30 seconds until you feel the muscle release. This technique can be uncomfortable but effective for releasing deeply held tension.

Cold and Heat Therapy for Acute and Chronic Pain:

Cold and heat therapy are often combined with massage for both acute and chronic pain relief. Cold therapy is particularly useful for reducing inflammation in the early stages of injury, while heat therapy promotes relaxation and increases blood flow to promote healing.

- **Cold Therapy:** Apply cold compresses or ice packs to the affected area for 15-20 minutes to reduce swelling and numb pain. This is particularly helpful for new injuries, sprains, or muscle strains.

- **Heat Therapy:** After the initial inflammation subsides, heat therapy can be used to relax muscles, increase circulation, and relieve pain. Use a warm towel or heating pad to apply heat to sore or stiff muscles, especially after exercise or during recovery from an injury.

Working with Athletes: Pre-Event, Post-Event, and Recovery Massages

Massage therapy is especially beneficial for athletes, whether they're professional athletes or simply people who enjoy sports and physical activity. Massage can help prevent injuries, improve performance, and speed up recovery—making it an essential part of any athlete's training routine.

Pre-Event Massage for Performance Enhancement:

A pre-event massage focuses on preparing the body for physical activity. The goal is to warm up the muscles, increase blood flow, and improve flexibility, which helps reduce the risk of injury. A pre-event massage is typically light and brisk, designed to invigorate the muscles without tiring them out.

- **Effleurage** is used to gently warm up the muscles.

- **Petrissage** can be applied lightly to increase circulation in the larger muscle groups that will be used in the event.

- **Stretching** helps lengthen the muscles, improving flexibility and range of motion.

This type of massage should be done 30-60 minutes before the event and is particularly helpful for athletes who engage in high-intensity activities like running, cycling, or competitive sports.

Post-Event Massage for Recovery and Relaxation:

After an event, muscles are often fatigued and tight. A post-event massage helps reduce muscle soreness, flush out lactic acid, and promote relaxation. This massage is typically deeper and slower, focusing on releasing built-up tension in the muscles.

- **Petrissage** is used to knead and release muscle tension.

- **Friction** can be applied to specific areas of tightness or soreness.

- **Stretching** is incorporated to keep muscles flexible and reduce post-event stiffness.

Post-event massage helps reduce recovery time, allowing the athlete to perform at their best in subsequent training sessions or events.

Recovery Massage for Long-Term Healing:

After the initial recovery phase, athletes often continue to benefit from regular recovery massages. This helps maintain muscle health, prevent injury, and reduce the chance of long-term issues.

- **Deep Tissue Massage** helps with persistent soreness and tightness that may remain after events.

- **Myofascial Release** and **Trigger Point Therapy** address deeper areas of tension and promote full muscle recovery.

- **Hydration and Stretching** should be combined with massage to promote overall muscle health.

By tailoring your approach to the individual athlete and the timing of their training or event, you can provide massages that promote optimal performance, injury prevention, and long-term recovery.

Conclusion

Massage is a powerful tool in the realm of pain relief and rehabilitation. Whether you're addressing chronic pain, aiding in injury recovery, or supporting an athlete's performance, the techniques in this chapter are vital for providing relief and encouraging healing. From using effleurage and petrissage to help with muscle soreness, to applying myofascial release for injury rehabilitation, massage can accelerate the body's natural healing process and bring comfort to those suffering from pain.

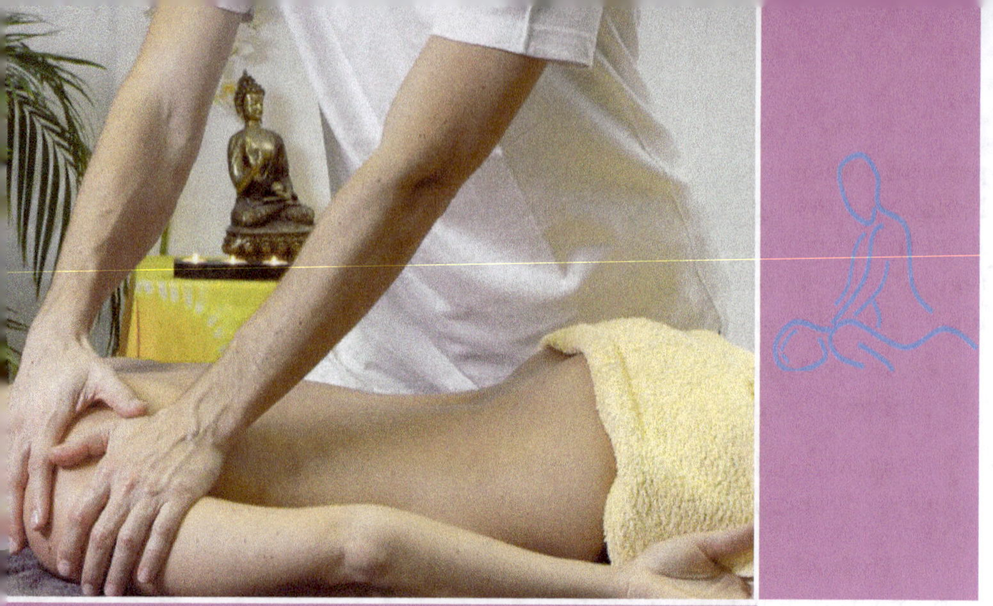

7

SWEDISH MASSAGE

WHAT YOU'LL LEARN

◊ WHAT IS SWEDISH MASSAGE?

◊ STEP-BY-STEP SWEDISH MASSAGE

◊ BENEFITS OF SWEDISH MASSAGE

Swedish massage is one of the most well-known and widely practiced forms of therapeutic massage. It is often the first choice for those seeking a relaxing, soothing experience, as it helps to calm both the body and mind. This form of massage is designed to enhance circulation, reduce stress, alleviate muscle tension, and promote overall wellness.

In this chapter, we'll explore the benefits of Swedish massage, its techniques, and how it can be used to promote both physical and emotional well-being. Whether you're looking for a way to relax after a stressful day, recover from muscle fatigue, or simply unwind, Swedish massage offers a gentle yet effective approach to healing.

What is Swedish Massage?

Swedish massage is a therapeutic massage technique that uses long, flowing strokes, kneading, and circular movements on the outer layers of muscles. The primary goal of Swedish massage is relaxation, but it also works to improve circulation, increase flexibility, and reduce muscle tension. Unlike deeper forms of massage (such as deep tissue massage), Swedish massage focuses on light to medium pressure and rhythmic movements, which allow the body to relax without feeling overwhelmed.

Swedish massage can be particularly beneficial for individuals who are new to massage therapy or those looking for a lighter, more soothing experience. It is also often recommended for stress relief, as it can promote the release of endorphins, the body's natural "feel-good" hormones, and reduce cortisol levels, the hormone associated with stress.

Step-by-Step Swedish Massage Guide

This step-by-step guide outlines how to perform a Swedish massage effectively.

Preparation

1. **Set Up the Space:**

   - Create a calm, comfortable environment. Dim the lights and play soft, soothing music.

   - Ensure the room is warm enough for relaxation.

2. **Gather Supplies:**

- Use a sturdy massage table or surface.

- Prepare massage oil or lotion to reduce friction on the skin.

3. Prepare Yourself:

- Wash your hands thoroughly.

- Remove any jewelry and keep your nails short to prevent scratching.

4. Position the Client:

- Ask the client to lie face down on the massage table with a pillow or bolster under their ankles for comfort.

Step 1: Effleurage (Warm-Up Strokes)

Effleurage consists of long, gliding strokes that warm up the muscles and increase circulation.

1. Apply Oil:

- Warm the massage oil in your hands and gently spread it over the client's back.

2. Perform Long Strokes:

- Use the flat part of your hands or fingertips to glide smoothly along the length of the back. Start at the lower back and move upward toward the shoulders.

- Apply light to medium pressure, adjusting based on the client's comfort.

3. Focus on Rhythm:

- Maintain a steady rhythm to promote relaxation.

- Repeat the strokes several times to evenly distribute the oil and prepare the muscles.

Step 2: Petrissage (Kneading Movements)

Petrissage involves kneading and lifting the muscles to release tension and improve flexibility.

1. Start with Large Muscle Groups:

- Using your hands, gently knead the muscles in the upper back and shoulders.

- Squeeze and lift the muscles as if kneading dough, then release.

2. **Vary Your Techniques:**

   • Use your thumbs for small, circular motions in tighter areas.

   • Alternate between one-handed and two-handed kneading for different muscle groups.

3. **Adjust Pressure:**

   • Apply deeper pressure in areas with more tension, but always communicate with the client to ensure comfort.

Step 3: Friction (Targeted Pressure)

Friction techniques focus on breaking down adhesions (knots) and improving circulation in deeper layers of tissue.

1. **Identify Tight Areas:**

   • Feel for areas of muscle tension or stiffness, such as knots in the shoulders or lower back.

2. **Use Circular Movements:**

   • With your thumbs or fingertips, apply firm pressure and make small, circular motions over tight spots.

3. **Increase Pressure Gradually:**

   • Start with light pressure and gradually increase as the tissue warms up. Avoid sudden, deep pressure that could cause discomfort.

Step 4: Tapotement (Percussive Movements)

Tapotement involves rhythmic tapping or striking motions that stimulate the nerves and energize the body.

1. **Form Your Hands:**

   • Cup your hands slightly, or make loose fists.

2. **Apply Gentle Percussion:**

   • Lightly tap or drum along the back, shoulders, and legs.

   • Keep the movements brisk and rhythmic to avoid discomfort.

3. **Use Sparingly:**

   • Tapotement is invigorating, so use it toward the end of the massage or in areas where increased stimulation is desired.

Step 5: Vibration (Shaking Movements)
Vibration techniques help release tension and soothe nerves.
   1. Place Your Hands:

   • Rest your hands gently on a specific area, such as the lower back or thighs.

   2. Shake or Vibrate:

   • Use quick, gentle movements to create a vibrating effect in the muscles.

   • This technique is particularly effective for relaxing smaller areas or calming the nervous system.

Step 6: Focus on Specific Areas

Address any areas of concern the client may have, such as the neck, shoulders, or lower back.
   1. Neck and Shoulders:

   • Use your thumbs to apply circular pressure along the neck and shoulder blades.

   • Perform gentle upward strokes to relieve tension in these areas.

   2 Lower Back:

   • Use long, firm strokes along the lower back, followed by kneading to release tightness.

   3. Arms and Legs:

   • Glide your hands along the limbs with effleurage, then knead the muscles for deeper relaxation.

Step 7: Cool Down

   1. Return to Effleurage:

   • Use long, soothing strokes to calm the muscles and signal the end of the massage.

   2. Wipe Off Excess Oil:

   • Use a warm, damp towel to gently wipe away any excess oil, if needed.

   3. Encourage Relaxation:

   • Allow the client to rest for a few minutes before getting up. Offer water to help with hydration and detoxification.

Tips for a Great Swedish Massage

- **Communicate:** Always check in with the client about pressure and comfort.

- **Pace Yourself:** Move slowly and intentionally to maintain a relaxing flow.

- **Stay Relaxed:** Keep your own posture and breathing calm to transfer positive energy to the client.

Benefits of Swedish Massage

Swedish massage is much more than a relaxing treat; it offers a wide range of physical, emotional, and mental benefits. Here are some of the most notable benefits of Swedish massage:

1. Stress Reduction and Relaxation

The primary benefit of Swedish massage is stress relief. The gentle, rhythmic strokes help to calm the nervous system, release muscle tension, and promote a sense of overall relaxation. Swedish massage is known for its ability to lower cortisol (the stress hormone) and increase the production of endorphins, helping you feel more at ease, both physically and emotionally.

2. Improved Circulation

Swedish massage stimulates blood flow, which improves circulation throughout the body. Increased circulation ensures that muscles receive more oxygen and nutrients, which can enhance muscle performance and speed up recovery after exercise. It also helps in flushing out metabolic waste products, reducing swelling and improving the body's detoxification process.

3. Pain Relief and Muscle Tension

Whether caused by stress, poor posture, or overexertion, muscle tension can lead to discomfort and pain. Swedish massage works to release tight muscles and alleviate the discomfort associated with stiffness or soreness. By focusing on muscle groups that are tense, Swedish massage can help improve flexibility and range of motion, reducing discomfort in areas like the neck, shoulders, and lower back.

4. Improved Flexibility and Mobility

Swedish massage helps to improve flexibility by releasing muscle tension and increasing blood flow to the tissues. When muscles are more relaxed, they can move more freely, improving overall flexibility and mobility. This can be particularly helpful for individuals who experience tightness in their muscles or joints due to sedentary lifestyles, overuse, or stress.

5. Promotes Better Sleep
Regular Swedish massage sessions can also improve sleep quality. The calming effects of the massage help to activate the parasympathetic nervous system, which is responsible for the body's relaxation response. As a result, individuals who receive Swedish massage may find it easier to fall asleep, stay asleep, and enjoy a deeper, more restful night's sleep.

6. Emotional Wellness and Mental Clarity
Beyond the physical benefits, Swedish massage also provides emotional and mental wellness benefits. The act of receiving a massage allows individuals to disconnect from daily stresses, focus on the present moment, and clear their minds. It helps to create a peaceful, tranquil environment, which can improve mental clarity, reduce anxiety, and boost overall well-being.

When to Seek Swedish Massage
Swedish massage is ideal for people of all ages and fitness levels. It is an excellent option for those who are looking to relax and relieve stress, or for individuals who need relief from muscle tension, pain, or soreness. It's also beneficial for those recovering from illness or surgery, as the gentle techniques can help promote healing without overwhelming the body.
Some specific situations where Swedish massage may be especially beneficial include:

- After a stressful workday to relieve tension and unwind.

- For chronic muscle pain or discomfort in the neck, shoulders, or lower back.

- As part of a self-care routine to improve flexibility, circulation, and overall well-being.

- To enhance athletic performance by increasing mobility and reducing muscle tightness.

- For mental relaxation, helping to ease anxiety and promote emotional balance.

Conclusion

Swedish massage is one of the most popular and accessible forms of massage therapy. Its gentle, soothing techniques provide a wide range of physical and emotional benefits, from relieving muscle tension and improving circulation to reducing stress and promoting relaxation. Whether you're seeking relief from pain, improved flexibility, or simply a peaceful escape from the demands of everyday life, Swedish massage offers a therapeutic solution that nurtures both body and mind.

By incorporating Swedish massage into your wellness routine, you can enjoy the many benefits it offers, supporting your overall health and well-being. Whether performed by a professional therapist or as a self-care practice, Swedish massage can be a key tool in achieving a balanced and healthy lifestyle.

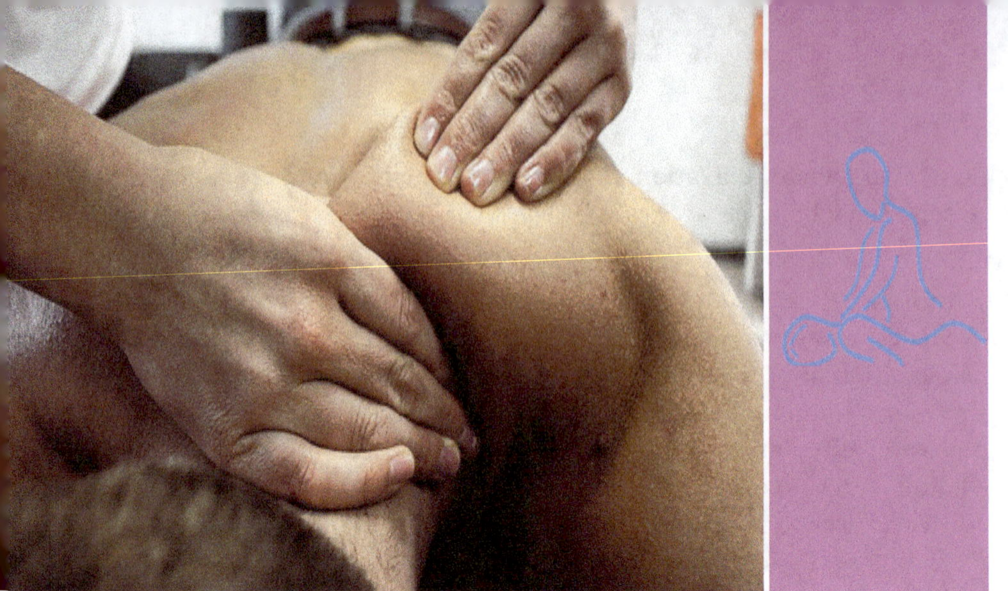

8

DEEP TISSUE MASSAGE

WHAT YOU'LL LEARN

◊ WHAT IS DEEP TISSUE MASSAGE?

◊ KEY TECHNIQUES IN DEEP TISSUE MASSAGE

◊ STEP-BY-STEP DEEP TISSUE MASSAGE

◊ BENEFITS OF DEEP TISSUE MASSAGE

Deep tissue massage is a therapeutic technique designed to release tension in the deeper layers of muscles and connective tissues. Unlike more superficial forms of massage, this approach focuses on areas of chronic pain, stiffness, and restricted movement. It's often used to address injuries, postural issues, and long-term muscular discomfort.

In this chapter, we'll explore what makes deep tissue massage unique, the benefits it offers, and how to apply its principles effectively. Whether you're a massage enthusiast or a practitioner looking to expand your skills, understanding deep tissue massage can be a valuable addition to your wellness toolkit.

What is Deep Tissue Massage?

Deep tissue massage is a methodical and slow approach that uses firm pressure to penetrate beyond the superficial muscles. It aims to address tension and adhesions (knots) in the deeper layers of muscle, fascia, and connective tissue. The technique involves sustained pressure and deliberate strokes, often using fingers, knuckles, forearms, or elbows.

This massage is ideal for individuals experiencing chronic pain or recovering from injuries, as it can help restore flexibility, relieve pain, and improve posture. It's particularly effective for conditions like lower back pain, sciatica, stiff necks, and shoulder tension caused by repetitive strain or stress.

Key Techniques in Deep Tissue Massage

1. Slow and Focused Strokes:

Deep tissue massage requires slow, deliberate movements that allow the therapist to penetrate deeply into the muscle layers. Common strokes include longitudinal gliding, kneading, and compression.

2. Sustained Pressure:

Applying consistent pressure to a specific area helps release knots and adhesions. Tools like elbows and knuckles are often used to maintain firm pressure.

3. Cross-Fiber Friction:

This technique involves moving across the muscle fibers rather than along their length. It's useful for breaking down scar tissue and increasing flexibility in stiff areas.

4. Muscle Stripping:

This involves running firm pressure along the length of a muscle, often with the thumb or forearm. It's effective for releasing tension and elongating tight muscles.

5. Trigger Point Therapy:

Trigger points, or areas of localized tension, are addressed by applying direct pressure until the tightness releases. This technique is often uncomfortable but highly effective for pain relief.

Step-by-Step Deep Tissue Massage Guide

Below is a step-by-step guide to performing Deep Tissue Massage effectively.

Preparation

1. **Set Up the Environment:**

   - Choose a quiet, warm space with minimal distractions.

   - Use a sturdy massage table or flat surface.

2. **Prepare the Tools:**

   - Use unscented or lightly scented oil or lotion to reduce friction and allow deeper strokes.

   - Have towels or a warm compress handy for comfort.

3. **Communicate with the Client:**

   - Discuss problem areas, pressure preferences, and medical history to tailor the massage.

   - Explain that deep tissue massage may involve some discomfort, but it should never be painful.

4. **Warm Your Hands:**

   - Rub your hands together or under warm water to make them comfortable before starting.

Step 1: Warm-Up with Light Strokes (Effleurage)

1. **Apply Oil:**

   • Warm the oil in your hands and gently spread it across the area you're working on.

2. **Use Long, Smooth Strokes:**

   • Begin with effleurage to warm up the muscles and improve circulation.

   • Glide your hands along the muscles using light to medium pressure to prepare the tissue for deeper work.

3. **Work Broadly:**

   • Cover large muscle groups like the back, thighs, or shoulders before focusing on smaller areas.

Step 2: Gradual Pressure with Kneading (Petrissage)

1. **Knead the Muscles:**

   • Use your thumbs, knuckles, or palms to knead the muscles in a rolling motion.

   • Work slowly to ensure that you reach deeper layers of muscle tissue without causing pain.

2. **Focus on Tense Areas:**

   • Pay extra attention to areas with knots or tightness, such as the shoulders, neck, or lower back.

   • Apply slightly firmer pressure in these areas while staying mindful of the client's comfort.

Step 3: Target Trigger Points

1. **Locate Trigger Points:**

   • Feel for areas of tightness or muscle knots. These points often feel harder than surrounding tissue.

   • Ask the client for feedback to identify particularly tender spots.

2. **Apply Sustained Pressure:**

   • Use your thumb, knuckle, or elbow to apply firm, sustained pressure to the trigger point.

- Hold the pressure for 10–30 seconds or until you feel the muscle release.

3. Encourage Relaxation:

- Ask the client to breathe deeply as you work on the trigger points. This helps the muscle relax and releases tension.

Step 4: Use Friction for Deeper Release

1. Apply Small, Circular Movements:

- With your fingertips or knuckles, make small, firm circles over tight areas.

- This technique breaks up adhesions and scar tissue in deeper layers of muscle.

3. Adjust the Pressure:

- Gradually increase pressure to reach deeper tissues but avoid causing pain.

- Work slowly and deliberately to avoid overwhelming the muscle.

Step 5: Work Along Muscle Fibers

Follow the Muscle's Direction:

- Use long, deep strokes along the length of the muscle fibers to stretch and realign them.

- For larger muscles like the back or thighs, use your forearms or elbows for sustained, deep pressure.

Cross-Fiber Work:

- Occasionally, use strokes that go across the muscle fibers to help break up knots and improve mobility.

Step 6: Focus on Specific Problem Areas

1. Neck and Shoulders:

- Use your thumbs to make small, firm circles along the base of the skull and down the neck.

- Apply deep, kneading strokes to the shoulders to release tension.

2. Lower Back:

- Use your forearm or elbow for long, deep strokes along the lumbar muscles.

- Be cautious with pressure to avoid discomfort in this sensitive area.

3. Legs and Thighs:

- Use your fists or forearms to work along the quadriceps and hamstrings.

- Apply deeper pressure to the calves, which often hold tension from standing or walking.

Step 7: Cool Down and Reassess

1. Return to Effleurage:

- Use light, flowing strokes to calm the muscles and signal the end of the session.

2. Wipe Off Excess Oil:

- Use a warm, damp towel to remove any remaining oil from the skin.

3. Encourage Rest:

- Allow the client to rest for a few minutes before getting up. Advise them to hydrate and avoid strenuous activity immediately after the massage.

Tips for Effective Deep Tissue Massage

- **Work Slowly:** Rushing can cause discomfort and reduce the effectiveness of deep tissue techniques.

- **Communicate Constantly:** Check in with the client about pressure and comfort throughout the session.

- **Use Your Body Weight:** Instead of relying solely on arm strength, use your body weight to apply deeper pressure without straining yourself.

- **Stay Mindful:** Be attentive to the client's body language and adjust your techniques as needed.

The Benefits of Deep Tissue Massage
1. Relieves Chronic Pain:
Deep tissue massage targets the root cause of chronic pain by breaking down adhesions and improving blood flow to affected areas. This can help alleviate pain caused by conditions like arthritis, fibromyalgia, and repetitive strain injuries.

2. Improves Mobility and Flexibility:
By releasing tight muscles and breaking up scar tissue, deep tissue massage enhances range of motion and flexibility. This is particularly beneficial for athletes or individuals recovering from surgeries or injuries.

3. Reduces Stress and Tension:
While deep tissue massage is more intense than other forms of massage, it still promotes relaxation by releasing endorphins and reducing stress hormones like cortisol. It's especially effective for those who hold tension in their bodies due to stress.

4. Speeds Recovery:
For athletes, deep tissue massage aids in post-workout recovery by reducing muscle soreness, improving circulation, and flushing out metabolic waste products like lactic acid. It also prepares the body for future physical activity by maintaining muscle health.

5. Enhances Posture and Alignment:
Poor posture often leads to muscle imbalances and chronic tension. Deep tissue massage helps correct these issues by loosening tight muscles and aligning connective tissues, resulting in better posture and reduced discomfort.

Who Can Benefit from Deep Tissue Massage?
1. Athletes:
Athletes often use deep tissue massage as part of their training regimen. It helps prevent injuries, speeds recovery, and maintains muscle health.

2. Individuals with Chronic Pain:
Those suffering from conditions like sciatica, lower back pain, or migraines often find relief through deep tissue techniques.

3. Desk Workers:

Long hours at a desk can lead to postural imbalances and chronic tension in the neck, shoulders, and back. Deep tissue massage can alleviate these issues and improve posture.

4. Recovery Patients:

People recovering from surgeries, injuries, or long-term immobility benefit from deep tissue massage as it helps break down scar tissue and restore mobility.

4. Monitor Feedback:

Regularly check in with the client to ensure the pressure is appropriate. Pain should always be tolerable, never overwhelming.

Conclusion

Deep tissue massage is a powerful tool for addressing chronic pain, improving mobility, and promoting overall well-being. While it requires patience and skill to perform effectively, the results are transformative for both the body and mind. Whether you're an athlete, a desk worker, or simply someone looking to release built-up tension, incorporating deep tissue massage into your wellness routine can lead to profound and lasting benefits.

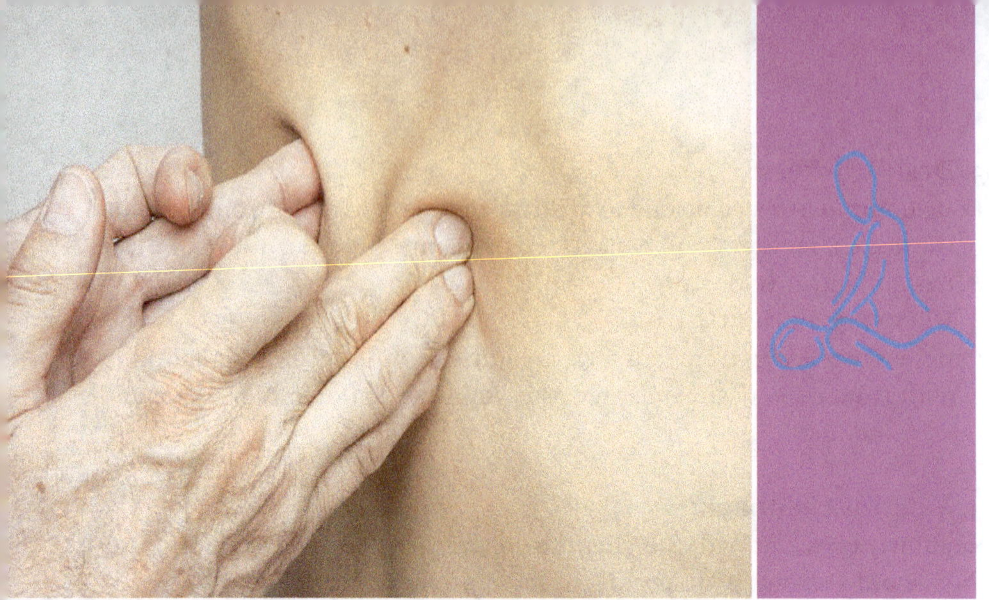

9

TRIGGER POINT THERAPY

 **WHAT YOU'LL LEARN** 

◊ WHAT ARE TRIGGER POINTS?

◊ TECHNIQUES FOR TRIGGER POINT THERAPY

◊ STEP-BY-STEP TRIGGER POINT THERAPY

◊ BENEFITS OF TRIGGER POINT THERAPY

◊ COMMON AREAS FOR TRIGGER POINT THERAPY

Trigger Point Therapy is a specialized massage technique that focuses on identifying and releasing trigger points—specific areas of tension within the muscles that can cause pain, stiffness, and discomfort. These points, often referred to as "knots," can create localized pain or refer pain to other areas of the body. Trigger Point Therapy is highly effective for managing chronic pain, improving mobility, and addressing postural imbalances.

In this chapter, we'll explore the nature of trigger points, the benefits of this therapy, techniques for identifying and treating them, and how to incorporate trigger point work into your overall wellness routine.

What Are Trigger Points?

Trigger points are hyperirritable spots within a muscle or fascia. These areas of tension feel like small nodules or bands of tightness under the skin. Trigger points can develop due to stress, overuse, poor posture, or injuries and can remain dormant for years until aggravated by physical or emotional strain.

Trigger points are categorized into two types:

- **Active Trigger Points:** These cause immediate pain, often felt as a deep ache, sharp sting, or burning sensation. Pain may be localized or referred to another part of the body. For example, a trigger point in the neck may cause headaches or jaw pain.

- **Latent Trigger Points:** These do not cause pain until pressure is applied. However, they can restrict movement and weaken the muscle, contributing to stiffness or fatigue.

Techniques for Trigger Point Therapy

1. Locating Trigger Points:

Finding a trigger point often involves palpating the muscle for areas of tightness, tenderness, or knots. These points may feel firm or rope-like under the fingers. The client might also feel a referral pattern of pain in a different area when the trigger point is pressed.

2. Applying Sustained Pressure:

Once a trigger point is located, sustained pressure is applied using the fingers, thumbs, knuckles, or elbows. The pressure should be firm but not unbearable, and it is held for 20–60 seconds. This pressure disrupts the cycle of tension and pain, encouraging the muscle to relax.

3. Using Ischemic Compression:
This involves applying steady, firm pressure to the trigger point until the muscle relaxes. The initial discomfort often gives way to a release, signaled by a decrease in pain or a feeling of warmth in the area.

4. Stretching After Release:
After the trigger point is released, gently stretching the muscle helps reinforce the relaxation and prevents the trigger point from reforming. For example, stretching the hamstrings after releasing a trigger point in the thigh can improve flexibility and comfort.

5. Self-Trigger Point Therapy:
Using tools like foam rollers, massage balls, or even a tennis ball, individuals can perform self-care to address trigger points in hard-to-reach areas. For example, rolling a ball against a wall to target the shoulder blade muscles is a common technique.

Step-by-Step Trigger Point Therapy Guide
Below is a step-by-step guide to performing deep Trigger Point Therapy effectively.

Preparation

1. **Create a Comfortable Environment:**

   - Ensure a quiet, warm, and calm space to help the person relax.

   - Use a sturdy massage table or chair that supports proper positioning.

2. **Prepare Supplies:**

   - Have massage oil or lotion available, though minimal use is needed for trigger point work to maintain grip on the skin.

3. **Communicate with the Client:**

   - Discuss the areas of pain or tension they are experiencing.

   - Explain the therapy may cause mild discomfort but should not be overly painful.

4. Warm Your Hands:

- Rub your hands together to ensure they are warm and comfortable to the touch.

Step 1: Warm Up the Muscles

Before targeting specific trigger points, it's important to warm up the surrounding muscles to reduce sensitivity and make the tissue more pliable.

1. Apply Light Strokes:

- Use gentle effleurage (long, gliding strokes) to warm the area.

- Cover the general region of the suspected trigger points, such as the shoulders, back, or legs.

2. Use Gentle Kneading:

- Apply light petrissage (kneading) to increase circulation and loosen the muscles.

Step 2: Locate the Trigger Points

Trigger points are small, tight knots or sensitive spots within the muscle tissue.

1. Palpate the Area:

- Use your fingers or thumbs to feel for small, tight nodules or areas of tension.

- Move slowly and press gently to identify points that feel harder or denser than surrounding tissue.

2. Confirm Trigger Points:

- Ask the client if they feel localized pain or referred pain in another area when pressure is applied.

- Referred pain is a key indicator of a trigger point.

Step 3: Apply Sustained Pressure

Once you locate a trigger point, use focused pressure to release it.

1. Position Your Thumb or Finger:

- Use your thumb, fingertips, knuckles, or a massage tool to apply pressure directly on the trigger point.

2. Apply Firm Pressure:

- Start with moderate pressure and gradually increase to a firm but tolerable level.

- Hold the pressure for 20–60 seconds or until you feel the muscle release or soften.

3. Encourage Relaxation:

- Ask the client to take deep, slow breaths.

- Remind them to relax the area as much as possible while you work.

Step 4: Use Circular or Cross-Fiber Movements

To further release tension, incorporate friction techniques around the trigger point.

1. Circular Motions:

- Make small, firm circles over the trigger point using your thumb or fingertips.

- This technique helps break up adhesions and improve blood flow.

2. Cross-Fiber Friction:

- Apply pressure perpendicular to the muscle fibers, moving back and forth.

- This can help reduce scar tissue and restore muscle elasticity.

Step 5: Reassess the Trigger Point

After working on the trigger point, check for progress.

1. Re-Palpate the Area:

- Gently press on the area to see if the tightness or pain has diminished.

- Ask the client if they feel any improvement.

2. Repeat if Necessary:

- If the trigger point is still active, repeat the process of applying pressure and using circular or cross-fiber techniques.

Step 6: Stretch the Muscle

Stretching helps realign the muscle fibers and prevents the trigger point from reactivating.

1. **Passive Stretching:**

- Gently move the client's limb to stretch the affected muscle.

- For example, stretch the hamstring after releasing trigger points in the thigh.

2. **Encourage Active Stretching:**

- Teach the client simple stretches they can do at home to maintain flexibility and prevent recurrence.

Step 7: Cool Down

1. **Use Light Strokes:**

- Return to gentle effleurage to relax the muscle and improve circulation.

- This also helps signal the end of the session.

2. **Apply a Warm Compress:**

- Place a warm towel over the treated area to soothe the muscle and encourage further relaxation.

Tips for Effective Trigger Point Therapy

- **Work Slowly:** Take your time to locate and release trigger points without rushing.

- **Communicate Frequently:** Regularly check in with the client about their comfort level and pain threshold.

- **Use Body Mechanics:** Maintain proper posture and use your body weight to apply pressure, reducing strain on your hands.

- **Hydration:** Advise the client to drink water after the session to flush out toxins released from the muscles.

The Benefits of Trigger Point Therapy

1. **Pain Relief:**

Trigger Point Therapy targets the source of pain rather than just the symptoms. Releasing a trigger point can alleviate chronic pain, including headaches, backaches, and joint discomfort.

2. **Improved Mobility:**

By reducing tension in tight muscles, Trigger Point Therapy restores flexibility and range of motion, making daily activities easier and more comfortable.

3. Stress Reduction:

Muscle tension is often linked to stress. Releasing trigger points helps relax the body, reducing the physical manifestations of stress and promoting emotional well-being.

4. Enhanced Circulation:

Releasing trigger points improves blood flow to the affected area, aiding in the delivery of nutrients and the removal of waste products, which accelerates healing.

5. Better Posture:

Persistent muscle tension can pull the body out of alignment. Addressing trigger points helps correct these imbalances, improving posture and reducing strain on joints and ligaments.

Common Areas for Trigger Point Therapy

Trigger points can develop anywhere in the body, but they are most common in areas subjected to stress and overuse. Here are some frequent locations:

- **Neck and Shoulders:** Trigger points here often cause tension headaches, neck pain, and stiffness.

- **Upper Back:** Tightness in the trapezius and rhomboid muscles can lead to shoulder pain or poor posture.

- **Lower Back:** Trigger points in the lumbar region often contribute to back pain and reduced mobility.

- **Hips and Glutes:** Points in these areas can cause sciatica-like symptoms, hip discomfort, or difficulty walking.

- **Legs and Feet:** Calf and foot trigger points can lead to plantar fasciitis or limited ankle flexibility.

Conclusion

Trigger Point Therapy is a powerful tool for relieving pain, improving mobility, and enhancing overall well-being. By addressing the root causes of tension and discomfort, this technique offers long-term benefits that go beyond temporary relief. Whether practiced by a professional or used as part of a self-care routine, Trigger Point Therapy empowers individuals to take control of their physical health and find relief from the daily burdens of stress and pain.

Understanding the principles and techniques of Trigger Point Therapy can transform how you care for your body, helping you live a healthier, more comfortable life.

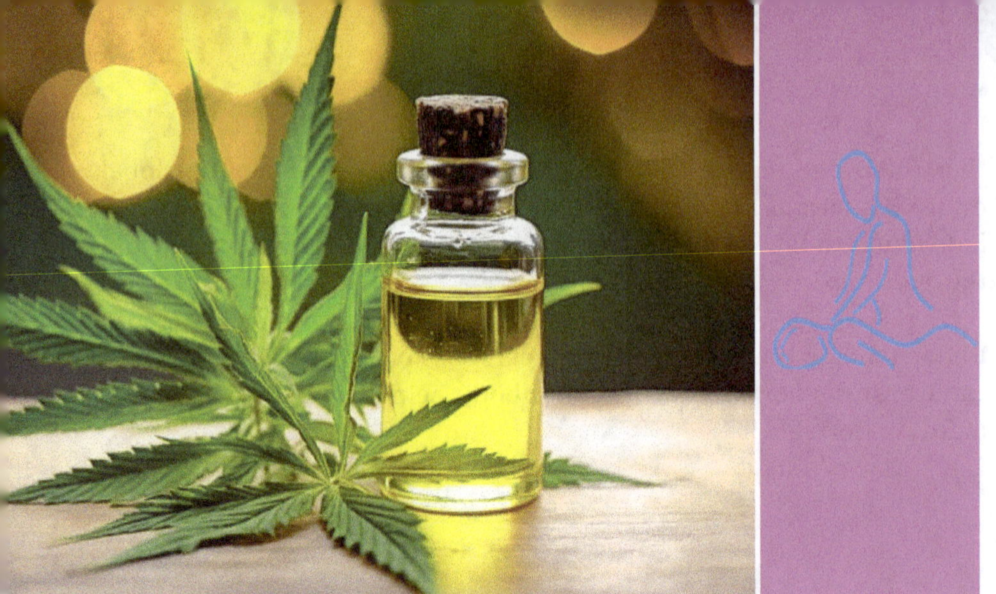

10

AROMATHERAPY MASSAGE

WHAT YOU'LL LEARN

◊ WHAT IS AROMATHERAPY MASSAGE?

◊ STEP-BY-STEP AROMATHERAPY MASSAGE

◊ BENEFITS OF AROMATHERAPY MASSAGE

Aromatherapy massage combines the therapeutic benefits of massage with the healing power of essential oils. This holistic approach works not only on the physical body but also on the mind and emotions. The use of carefully selected essential oils during a massage can enhance the experience by providing soothing scents that promote relaxation, reduce stress, and support overall wellness.

In this chapter, we'll explore what aromatherapy massage is, the benefits of using essential oils during a massage, how to incorporate them into your practice, and which oils are most commonly used for various therapeutic effects. Whether you are looking to unwind after a long day, improve your mood, or address physical discomfort, aromatherapy massage offers a natural and holistic approach to healing.

What is Aromatherapy Massage?

Aromatherapy massage is a therapeutic treatment that involves the use of essential oils—concentrated plant extracts—applied to the skin through massage techniques. These oils are known for their ability to affect both the mind and body, influencing mood, reducing tension, and promoting relaxation.

The massage techniques used in aromatherapy are similar to those in Swedish or other relaxing massages, with the added benefit of aromatic oils. The combination of touch and scent creates a deeply relaxing experience that can address both physical and emotional issues.

Essential oils are typically mixed with a carrier oil, such as coconut or almond oil, to dilute them and make them safe for skin application. As the therapist applies the oil through massage, the scent molecules are absorbed through the skin and into the bloodstream, while the aroma is inhaled into the lungs. The mind and body respond to both the physical touch and the fragrance, creating a holistic healing experience.

The Power of Essential Oils

Essential oils are the natural, aromatic compounds extracted from plants, flowers, seeds, and herbs. Each oil has a unique chemical composition that gives it distinct therapeutic properties. When used in aromatherapy massage, essential oils help to:

- **Promote relaxation and stress relief:** Many essential oils have calming effects that can help reduce anxiety, ease tension, and promote a peaceful state of mind.

- **Alleviate physical discomfort:** Certain oils are known to have analgesic or anti-inflammatory properties, making them effective for muscle pain, joint discomfort, and headaches.

- **Boost mood and emotional well-being:** Scents such as lavender, rose, and citrus are known for their uplifting and mood-enhancing effects.

- **Support immune function:** Some oils have antimicrobial or antibacterial properties that help support the immune system and protect against illness.

- **Enhance skin health:** Some essential oils are great for improving the appearance and health of the skin, reducing acne, dryness, or signs of aging.

Essential oils can be used for different purposes based on their individual properties. For example, lavender is commonly used for relaxation, while peppermint may be used to relieve headaches or digestive discomfort. Some oils can also be blended to create a synergistic effect, amplifying their therapeutic properties.

Step-by-Step Aromatherapy Massage Guide

Here's a step-by-step guide to performing an aromatherapy massage.

Preparation

1. **Choose Essential Oils:**

- Select essential oils based on the needs or preferences of the recipient.

  - **Lavender:** Relaxation and stress relief.

  - **Eucalyptus:** Respiratory support and muscle relief.

  - **Peppermint:** Energy boost and pain relief.

  - **Chamomile:** Calming and anti-inflammatory effects.

- Ensure the oils are high quality, pure, and safe for skin use.

2. Dilute the Essential Oils:

- Mix 5–10 drops of essential oil with 1 ounce (30 ml) of carrier oil (e.g., coconut, jojoba, almond, or grapeseed oil). This prevents skin irritation and ensures even application.

3. Create a Relaxing Environment:

- Dim the lights and play calming music.

- Use an oil diffuser or light a candle to enhance the ambiance.

4. Warm Your Hands:

- Rub your hands together to ensure they're warm and comfortable before touching the recipient.

5. Communicate with the Recipient:

- Ask about allergies, sensitivities, and any areas of tension or pain to tailor the massage accordingly.

Step 1: Begin with Light Effleurage

1. Apply the Oil Blend:

- Warm a small amount of the diluted essential oil in your hands.

- Gently spread it over the recipient's skin using long, gliding strokes (effleurage) to warm up the muscles and distribute the oil evenly.

2. Focus on Relaxation:

- Start with light pressure to allow the recipient to acclimate to your touch and the scent of the oils.

- Cover large areas like the back, legs, or arms to promote relaxation and circulation.

Step 2: Gradually Build Pressure

1. Use Kneading Movements (Petrissage):

- Knead the muscles in a rolling motion, working slowly to release tension.

- Focus on areas prone to stress, such as the shoulders, neck, and lower back.

2. Incorporate Breathing Cues:

• Encourage the recipient to take deep breaths, inhaling the aroma of the essential oils.

• Match your movements to their breathing rhythm for a more synchronized experience.

Step 3: Work on Specific Areas
1. Back and Shoulders:

• Use your thumbs to make circular motions along the shoulders and spine.

• Apply medium pressure to release knots while avoiding direct pressure on the spine itself.

2. Arms and Hands:

• Use light strokes from the shoulders down to the hands.

• Massage the palms and fingers individually, applying gentle pressure to relieve tension.

3. Legs and Feet:

• Start at the thighs and work down to the feet, using long strokes to relax the muscles.

• Focus on the calves and soles of the feet, which often carry stress.

• Incorporate reflexology techniques on the feet for added therapeutic benefit.

Step 4: Integrate Aromatherapy Techniques
1. Inhalation:

• Encourage the recipient to deeply inhale the aroma by placing your hands near their face for a few seconds.

• This enhances the emotional and psychological effects of the essential oils.

2. Apply to Key Points:

• Use extra oil to massage pulse points such as the temples, wrists, and behind the ears.

- These areas are particularly receptive to the benefits of aromatherapy.

Step 5: Incorporate Gentle Stretching

1. Stretch the Limbs:

- Gently stretch the arms, legs, or neck to improve flexibility and reduce tension.

- Keep the movements slow and mindful to avoid discomfort.

2. Align Movements with Relaxation:

- Use stretching as a transition to more relaxing techniques as the session progresses.

Step 6: Cool Down and Reassess

1. Return to Light Effleurage:

- Use soft, flowing strokes to signal the end of the session and soothe the muscles.

- Ensure that the oil is fully absorbed into the skin.

2. Check in with the Recipient:

- Ask how they feel and if there are any areas that need additional attention.

Step 7: Provide Aftercare Tips

1. Hydrate:

- Advise the recipient to drink water after the massage to flush out toxins released during the session.

2. Rest and Reflect:

- Encourage relaxation and mindfulness to extend the benefits of the massage.

3. Essential Oil Care:

- Recommend using similar essential oils in diffusers or baths to continue the therapeutic effects at home.

Tips for Effective Aromatherapy Massage

- **Choose Oils Carefully:** Avoid using essential oils on individuals with allergies, sensitivities, or during pregnancy without professional guidance.

- **Monitor Pressure:** Adjust pressure based on the recipient's comfort, keeping the session soothing rather than overly intense.

- **Pace Yourself:** Slow, deliberate movements maximize the calming and healing effects of both the massage and the aromatherapy.

Benefits of Aromatherapy Massage

1. Reduces Stress and Anxiety:

One of the most significant benefits of aromatherapy massage is its ability to reduce stress. The combination of soothing touch and calming scents triggers the parasympathetic nervous system, which is responsible for the "rest and digest" response. This helps to lower cortisol levels (the stress hormone) and encourage relaxation. Lavender, chamomile, and bergamot are especially well-known for their stress-reducing properties.

2. Improves Sleep Quality:

Many people struggle with insomnia or disrupted sleep patterns due to stress, anxiety, or physical discomfort. Aromatherapy massage can be an effective tool for improving sleep. The calming effects of oils like lavender, frankincense, and ylang-ylang promote deep relaxation and help the body prepare for restful sleep. Aromatherapy can also address underlying issues like muscle tension, which can contribute to difficulty sleeping.

3. Alleviates Muscle and Joint Pain:

Aromatherapy massage is particularly helpful for those suffering from muscle aches, stiffness, or joint pain. Essential oils like peppermint, eucalyptus, and rosemary have analgesic and anti-inflammatory properties, which can soothe sore muscles, relieve tension, and improve circulation. These oils can be massaged into the muscles and joints to provide relief from discomfort caused by exercise, stress, or injury.

4. Improves Mood and Emotional Wellness:

The use of essential oils can have a profound effect on emotional health. The sense of smell is directly linked to the limbic system, the part of the brain that regulates emotions. Scents like citrus (e.g., lemon, orange), rose, and jasmine are uplifting and help to reduce feelings of sadness or irritability. A session of aromatherapy massage can elevate mood, reduce anxiety, and promote a sense of joy and well-being.

5. Enhances Skin Health:

In addition to the emotional and physical benefits, aromatherapy massage can support skin health. Essential oils such as tea tree, lavender, and geranium have antibacterial properties that help cleanse and rejuvenate the skin. Oils like rosehip and frankincense are known for their ability to reduce the appearance of scars, wrinkles, and age spots, while promoting healthy, glowing skin.

6. Boosts Immune Function:

Aromatherapy massage can also help to strengthen the immune system. Oils like eucalyptus, tea tree, and thyme have antimicrobial properties that can help protect the body from illness and support overall immune health. These oils help to stimulate the immune system, cleanse the airways, and promote general wellness.

Common Essential Oils Used in Aromatherapy Massage

There are many essential oils available, each with unique benefits. Here are some of the most commonly used oils in aromatherapy massage:

- **Lavender:** Known for its calming and soothing properties, lavender is often used to reduce stress, promote relaxation, and improve sleep.

- **Peppermint:** Cooling and invigorating, peppermint is great for relieving muscle pain, headaches, and digestive discomfort.

- **Eucalyptus:** Often used to treat respiratory issues, eucalyptus helps to clear the sinuses, promote deep breathing, and reduce muscle pain.

- **Rosemary:** A stimulating oil that helps to improve circulation, relieve tension, and support mental clarity.

- **Chamomile:** Calming and soothing, chamomile is used to alleviate stress, reduce anxiety, and support skin health.

- **Bergamot:** Known for its mood-boosting effects, bergamot helps to reduce anxiety and elevate mood.

- **Tea Tree:** A powerful antibacterial oil that helps cleanse the skin and support the immune system.

- **Frankincense:** Grounding and calming, frankincense helps to relieve stress, promote relaxation, and improve skin tone.

- **Geranium:** Balancing and rejuvenating, geranium is beneficial for skin health, hormonal balance, and emotional wellness.

Conclusion

Aromatherapy massage offers a unique and holistic way to promote relaxation, reduce stress, and support overall health and wellness. By combining the therapeutic power of touch with the healing properties of essential oils, this massage technique addresses both physical and emotional concerns. Whether you are looking to relieve muscle tension, improve sleep, uplift your mood, or enhance skin health, aromatherapy massage provides a natural and effective approach to self-care.

By incorporating essential oils into your massage practice, you can create a deeply relaxing and therapeutic experience that nurtures the body, mind, and spirit. Whether you are a professional massage therapist or someone looking to incorporate aromatherapy into your personal wellness routine, aromatherapy massage can be a powerful tool for healing and relaxation.

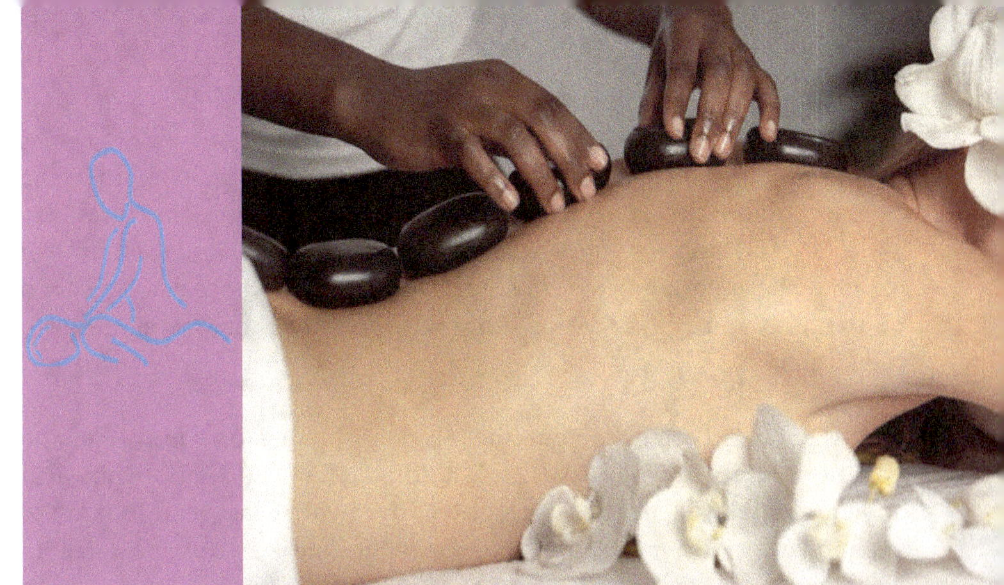

11

HOT STONE MASSAGE

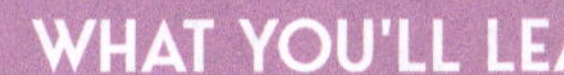

WHAT YOU'LL LEARN

◇ THE ORIGINS OF HOT STONE MASSAGE

◇ TECHNIQUES IN HOT STONE MASSAGE

◇ STEP-BY-STEP HOT STONE MASSAGE

◇ BENEFITS OF HOT STONE MASSAGE

◇ TOOLS AND MATERIALS FOR HOT STONE

MASSAGE

Hot stone massage is a therapeutic technique that combines the soothing properties of heated stones with traditional massage methods. The stones, typically made of basalt—a volcanic rock known for its heat-retention properties—are warmed and strategically placed on the body to release tension, improve circulation, and promote deep relaxation.

In this chapter, we'll explore the origins of hot stone massage, the benefits it offers, and how to use this method effectively for both physical and emotional well-being. Whether you're new to massage or looking to expand your skills, mastering hot stone techniques can provide a deeply enriching experience.

The Origins of Hot Stone Massage

The practice of using heated stones for healing dates back thousands of years. Ancient cultures, including those in China, India, and the Americas, used hot stones in rituals and therapies to ease muscle pain, improve energy flow, and detoxify the body.

Modern hot stone massage was popularized in the 1990s, blending ancient techniques with contemporary massage practices. Today, it's a staple in spas and wellness centers worldwide, renowned for its ability to provide profound relaxation and therapeutic benefits.

Techniques in Hot Stone Massage

1. Placement:

- Begin by placing heated stones on key areas of the body, such as the back, shoulders, and legs. These areas hold tension and benefit most from the warmth.

- Allow the heat to penetrate for a few minutes before beginning the massage.

2. Gliding Movements:

- Use stones to perform long, sweeping strokes along the muscles. This combines the benefits of traditional massage with the soothing effects of heat.

- Adjust pressure and pace based on the recipient's preferences.

3. Targeted Pressure:

- For knots or trigger points, use smaller stones to apply gentle pressure to release tension.

- Circular movements can help address localized tightness.

4. Cooling Stones:

- Alternating hot and cold stones can stimulate circulation and provide relief for inflammation or swelling.

5. Hand-Free Techniques:

- For experienced practitioners, hot stones can be used as an extension of the hands, applying heat and pressure simultaneously for deeper muscle work.

Step-by-Step Hot Stone Massage Guide

Below is a step-by-step guide to performing a hot stone massage.

Preparation

1. **Gather Supplies:**

- **Hot Stones:** Basalt stones are commonly used because they retain heat well. Have a variety of sizes for different body areas.

- **Heating Equipment:** Use a professional stone heater to warm the stones. Avoid using a microwave or stovetop as this can lead to uneven heating and potential burns.

- **Massage Oil:** Use a light, non-greasy oil to allow smooth gliding of the stones.

2. **Prepare the Environment:**

- Create a quiet, calming atmosphere with soft lighting and relaxing music.

- Ensure the room is warm, as the recipient will be partially uncovered during the massage.

3. **Heat the Stones:**

- Warm the stones to a temperature between 120–130°F (49–54°C).

- Test the stones on your forearm or wrist to ensure they are comfortably warm, not hot.

4. Communicate with the Client:

- Discuss any areas of tension or discomfort and ensure the recipient is comfortable with the use of heated stones.

Step 1: Prepare the Body
1. Apply Oil:

- Begin by applying a thin layer of massage oil to the recipient's skin.

- This helps the stones glide smoothly and prevents skin irritation.

2. Warm the Muscles:

- Use light effleurage (gliding strokes) with your hands to prepare the muscles for the heat.

Step 2: Place the Stones
1. Stationary Placement:

- Place warm stones on key areas of the body to promote relaxation:

  - Along the spine.

  - On the shoulders.

  - On the palms of the hands or soles of the feet.

- Cover the stones with a towel to protect the skin from direct heat.

2. Leave for 5–10 Minutes:

- Allow the heat to penetrate the muscles while you massage other areas or prepare for the next step.

Step 3: Massage with the Stones
1. Hold the Stones Properly:

- Use one or two stones in your hands to perform the massage.

- Grip the stones firmly but gently to maintain control.

2. Use Long, Gliding Strokes:

- Glide the stones along the muscles using effleurage techniques.

- Apply even pressure, adjusting based on the recipient's comfort level.

3. Focus on Tension Areas:

- Use smaller stones for precision work on areas like the neck, shoulders, and lower back.

- Combine heat with gentle pressure to release tension.

Step 4: Alternate with Manual Massage

1. Combine Hands and Stones:

- Alternate between massaging with the stones and using your hands to keep the session dynamic and personal.

2. Use Kneading Techniques:

- Knead the muscles with your hands to further loosen tension, especially after applying heat.

Step 5: Target Specific Areas

1. Back and Shoulders:

- Use medium-sized stones for long strokes along the spine and shoulder blades. Avoid direct pressure on the spine itself.

2. Arms and Hands:

- Use small stones to massage the arms, focusing on the forearms and palms.

- Place a warm stone in each hand for additional relaxation.

3. Legs and Feet:

- Glide larger stones along the thighs and calves.

- Use smaller stones for precise work on the feet and toes.

Step 6: Cool Down and Reassess

1. Remove Stationary Stones:

- Gently remove any stones left in place on the body.

2. Cool Down with Hands:

- Finish with light effleurage using your hands to relax the muscles and signal the end of the session.

3. Reassess the Client's Comfort:

- Ask the recipient how they feel and whether there are any areas that need additional attention.

Aftercare Tips

1. Encourage Hydration:

- Advise the client to drink water after the massage to flush out toxins released from the muscles.

2. Provide Recovery Advice:

- Suggest the client rest and avoid strenuous activity for the remainder of the day to allow their body to fully absorb the benefits.

Safety Tips

- **Avoid Direct Heat on Sensitive Areas:** Use extra caution on bony areas, sensitive skin, or areas with poor circulation.

- **Communicate Constantly:** Check in regularly with the recipient to ensure the heat and pressure are comfortable.

- **Check the Temperature:** Always test the stones on your wrist or arm before placing them on the client to ensure they're not too hot.

- **Protect the Skin:** Place a towel or cloth between the stone and the skin for individuals with sensitive skin or when using higher temperatures.

- **Avoid Certain Conditions:** Hot stone massage is not recommended for individuals with open wounds, skin conditions, diabetes, or circulatory disorders. Pregnant individuals and those with heat sensitivities should also avoid this therapy.

- **Stay Hydrated:** Encourage the recipient to drink water before and after the massage to support detoxification and hydration.

Benefits of Hot Stone Massage

1. Relieves Muscle Tension:

The heat from the stones penetrates deep into the muscles, promoting relaxation and easing tightness. This makes it especially beneficial for individuals with chronic pain or stiffness.

2. Enhances Circulation:
The warmth of the stones dilates blood vessels, improving blood flow and oxygen delivery to tissues. Enhanced circulation helps reduce inflammation and speeds up the healing process.

3. Promotes Relaxation:
Hot stone massage engages the parasympathetic nervous system, reducing stress and promoting a state of deep relaxation. This can help alleviate anxiety, improve sleep, and restore balance to the body.

4. Alleviates Pain and Discomfort:
Whether caused by injury, tension, or chronic conditions like arthritis, the targeted application of heat can reduce pain and improve mobility.

5. Detoxifies the Body:
The warmth stimulates the lymphatic system, encouraging the removal of toxins and waste products from the body.

Tools and Materials for Hot Stone Massage
1. The Stones:

- **Basalt Stones:** Preferred for their smooth texture and excellent heat retention.

- **Sizes and Shapes:** Larger stones are used for the back, thighs, and torso, while smaller ones are ideal for hands, feet, and face.

2. Heating Equipment:

- **Stone Warmer:** A professional-grade heater with adjustable temperature settings is ideal.

- **Water Temperature:** Stones should be heated to 120°F–130°F (49°C–54°C) to avoid burns.

3. Lubricants:
Using massage oils or creams helps the stones glide smoothly over the skin. Choose oils with relaxing scents, like lavender or chamomile, for added aromatherapy benefits.

4. Towels and Linens:
Towels or cloths are used to protect the skin from direct contact with overly hot stones and to clean and cool the stones during the session.

Conclusion

Hot stone massage is a versatile and deeply therapeutic technique that blends heat with the art of touch. It offers profound relaxation, relief from muscle tension, and enhanced circulation, making it an ideal practice for individuals seeking both physical and emotional healing.

Whether practiced professionally or as part of a personal wellness routine, hot stone massage is a powerful way to nurture the body and mind, providing warmth, comfort, and renewal.

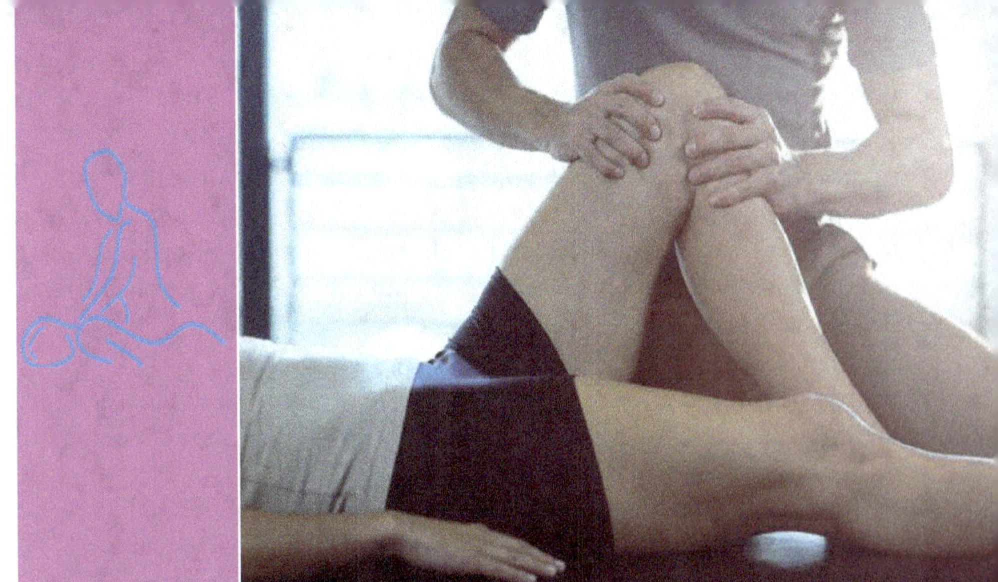

12

SPORTS MASSAGE

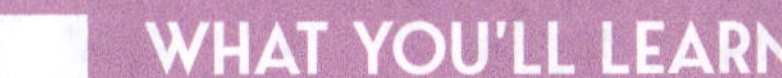

WHAT YOU'LL LEARN

◊ WHAT IS SPORTS MASSAGE?

◊ TYPES OF SPORTS MASSAGE

◊ TECHNIQUES USED IN SPORTS MASSAGE

◊ STEP-BY-STEP SPORTS MASSAGE

◊ BENEFITS OF SPORTS MASSAGE

◊ COMMON SPORTS RELATED ISSUES

ADDRESSED BY SPORTS MASSAGE

Sports massage is a specialized form of bodywork designed to optimize athletic performance, prevent injuries, and aid in recovery. It combines various techniques to address the specific needs of active individuals, whether they are professional athletes, fitness enthusiasts, or weekend warriors.

In this chapter, we'll explore the benefits of sports massage, its core techniques, and how it can be adapted to meet the unique demands of different sports and activities.

What is Sports Massage?

Sports massage focuses on the muscles, joints, and connective tissues that are most engaged during physical activity. Its primary goals include improving flexibility, reducing soreness, enhancing circulation, and promoting faster recovery. Unlike relaxation-focused massages, sports massage is dynamic and tailored to the athlete's needs before, during, or after physical exertion.

Types of Sports Massage

1. Pre-Event Massage:

- Designed to prepare the body for athletic performance.

- Focuses on warming up muscles, increasing circulation, and improving flexibility.

- Typically lighter and more stimulating, lasting 10–15 minutes.

2. Post-Event Massage:

- Helps the body recover after intense physical exertion.

- Emphasizes relaxation, reducing muscle soreness, and flushing out metabolic waste.

- Sessions usually last 20–30 minutes and focus on gentle, soothing techniques.

3. Maintenance Massage:

- Regular sessions designed to address muscle imbalances, prevent injuries, and maintain peak performance.

- Combines deep tissue work with stretching and range-of-motion exercises.

4. Rehabilitation Massage:

- Focuses on recovery from injuries such as sprains, strains, or overuse issues.

- Works alongside physical therapy to promote healing and regain function.

Techniques Used in Sports Massage
1. Effleurage:

- Long, gliding strokes are used to warm up the muscles, stimulate circulation, and prepare the body for deeper work.

- Typically applied at the beginning and end of a session.

2. Petrissage:

- Kneading and rolling movements help break up adhesions, increase blood flow, and release muscle tension.

3. Compression:

- Firm, rhythmic pressure applied to muscle groups improves circulation and prepares the body for strenuous activity.

4. Deep Tissue Techniques:

- Focused pressure is applied to deeper muscle layers, targeting specific areas of tension or tightness.

- Especially useful for addressing chronic pain or tightness.

5. Trigger Point Therapy:

- Identifies and releases specific points of tension in muscles that may cause pain or restrict movement.

6. Stretching:

- Passive and active stretching techniques enhance flexibility and reduce the risk of injury.

- Often combined with massage for a comprehensive approach.

Step-by-Step Sports Massage Guide
Here's a step-by-step guide to performing a general sports massage.

Preparation

1. Gather Supplies:

- **Massage Oil or Lotion:** Use a light, non-greasy product that allows smooth strokes without excessive slipperiness.

- **Towels or Linens:** To cover the recipient and ensure comfort.

- **A Comfortable Table or Chair:** Ensure the recipient can lie or sit in a supported position.

2. Create a Suitable Environment:

- Maintain a clean, professional, and well-lit space.

- Ensure the room is warm and free of distractions.

3. Communicate with the Recipient:

- Discuss their specific needs and areas of tension or soreness.

- Determine if the session is for pre-event preparation, post-event recovery, or general maintenance.

4. Understand Contraindications:

- Avoid massaging injured, inflamed, or swollen areas.

- Ensure the recipient is hydrated and has no medical conditions that could make massage unsafe.

Step 1: Begin with Light Effleurage

1. Apply Oil:

- Warm the oil in your hands and spread it evenly over the recipient's body.

- Use long, gliding strokes (effleurage) to warm up the muscles, promote circulation, and relax the recipient.

2. Focus on Large Muscle Groups:

- Start with broad strokes on areas such as the back, thighs, or calves.

- Gradually increase pressure to prepare the muscles for deeper work.

Step 2: Deep Tissue Techniques for Muscle Release

1. **Petrissage (Kneading):**

   - Use kneading techniques to work deeper into the muscles.

   - Focus on major muscle groups like the hamstrings, quadriceps, and shoulders.

2. **Compression:**

   - Apply rhythmic pressing and releasing with your palms or fists.

   - This technique increases circulation and prepares the muscles for intense activity.

3. **Stripping:**

   - Use your thumbs or forearms to apply firm, slow strokes along the length of the muscle fibers.

   - This helps release tension and elongate the muscles.

Step 3: Address Specific Muscle Groups

1. **Back and Shoulders:**

   - Use your thumbs to trace along the trapezius and rhomboid muscles.

   - Apply circular motions to release tension in the upper back.

2. **Legs:**

   - Work on the quadriceps and hamstrings with long, firm strokes.

   - Use deeper pressure on the calves to address tightness and improve flexibility.

3. **Arms and Hands:**

   - Massage the biceps and triceps with kneading movements.

   - Pay attention to the forearms, which are often tight in athletes who use their arms frequently.

4. **Feet:**

   - Focus on the soles and arches using your thumbs for precise pressure.

   - Stretch and massage the toes to improve flexibility and relieve

tension.

Step 4: Incorporate Stretching

1. Passive Stretching:

- Gently move the recipient's limbs through their range of motion to stretch the muscles.

- For example, bend the leg at the knee and gently press it toward the chest to stretch the hamstrings.

2. Active-Assisted Stretching:

- Encourage the recipient to actively engage in the stretch while you guide the movement.

- This enhances flexibility and prepares the muscles for activity.

Step 5: Use Trigger Point Therapy for Specific Issues

1. Identify Trigger Points:

- Look for knots or areas of tightness that cause referred pain.

- Common areas include the shoulders, neck, and lower back.

2. Apply Pressure:

- Use your thumb or knuckles to apply steady pressure to the trigger point.

- Hold for 10–30 seconds, gradually increasing the intensity as tolerated.

3. Release and Reassess:

- Slowly reduce pressure and ask the recipient how they feel.

- Repeat if needed, but avoid overworking a single area.

Step 6: Tailor Techniques Based on the Session Purpose

1. Pre-Event Massage:

- Use quick, stimulating strokes to energize the muscles.

- Avoid deep work to prevent soreness or fatigue.

- Focus on areas directly involved in the sport.

2. Post-Event Massage:

- Use slower, gentler techniques to relax the muscles and

promote recovery.

- Incorporate lymphatic drainage to reduce swelling and remove toxins.

3. Maintenance Massage:

- Combine deep tissue work and stretching to address chronic tension and improve flexibility.

- Focus on restoring balance to overused or strained muscles.

Step 7: Cool Down and Finish
Light Effleurage:

- Return to gentle, gliding strokes to relax the recipient and complete the session.

Stretching:

- End with a final round of stretching to leave the muscles feeling lengthened and loose.

Reassess:

- Ask the recipient how they feel and address any lingering tension areas.

Aftercare Tips
1. Encourage Hydration:

- Advise the recipient to drink plenty of water to flush out toxins released during the massage.

2. Rest and Recovery:

- Suggest light activity and rest to support recovery, especially after intense sports events.

3. Follow-Up:

- Recommend regular sports massages to maintain muscle health and prevent injuries.

Safety Tips

- Always adjust pressure based on the recipient's comfort.

- Avoid massaging injured or inflamed areas.

- Be mindful of contraindications, such as recent surgeries or medical conditions.

The Benefits of Sports Massage

1. Improves Performance:

Regular sports massage keeps muscles supple and flexible, enhancing an athlete's ability to perform at their peak.

2. Prevents Injuries:

By identifying and addressing muscle imbalances or tightness, sports massage reduces the risk of strains, sprains, and other injuries.

3. Speeds Up Recovery:

Post-event sports massage helps flush out lactic acid, reduce inflammation, and promote tissue repair, enabling athletes to recover faster after intense activity.

4. Relieves Pain and Tension:

Chronic muscle tension or soreness from repetitive movements can be alleviated with targeted massage techniques.

5. Enhances Flexibility and Range of Motion:

By loosening tight muscles and connective tissue, sports massage improves joint mobility and overall flexibility, critical for athletic performance.

Common Sports-Related Issues Addressed by Sports Massage

1. Muscle Soreness (DOMS):

Delayed onset muscle soreness (DOMS) is a common issue after intense exercise. Sports massage reduces discomfort by improving circulation and promoting tissue repair.

2. Tendon and Ligament Strain:

Gentle techniques help alleviate pain and promote healing for sprained or strained tendons and ligaments.

3. Overuse Injuries:

Repetitive motions can lead to conditions like tennis elbow or runner's knee. Sports massage targets affected areas to reduce inflammation and tension.

4. Postural Imbalances:
Improper posture during sports can lead to muscle strain. Massage helps correct these imbalances by releasing tight muscles and improving alignment.

5. Scar Tissue and Adhesions:
Massage techniques break down scar tissue, improving mobility and reducing discomfort after injuries.

Adapting Sports Massage to Different Activities

1. Runners:
Focus on the legs, hips, and lower back to address tightness in the hamstrings, calves, and glutes.
Stretching is often included to enhance flexibility and prevent injuries.

2. Cyclists:
Work on the lower back, quads, and neck to relieve tension caused by prolonged posture.
Deep tissue techniques help address tight muscles in the legs and hips.

3. Swimmers:
Target the shoulders, upper back, and arms to relieve strain from repetitive overhead movements.
Gentle techniques can improve flexibility and range of motion in the shoulders.

4. Weightlifters:
Focus on the back, shoulders, and arms to address tightness and improve muscle recovery.
Trigger point therapy helps release tension in overworked areas.

Conclusion

Sports massage is a powerful tool for enhancing athletic performance, speeding up recovery, and preventing injuries. By addressing the unique needs of active individuals, this specialized technique provides a pathway to peak physical condition and long-term wellness.

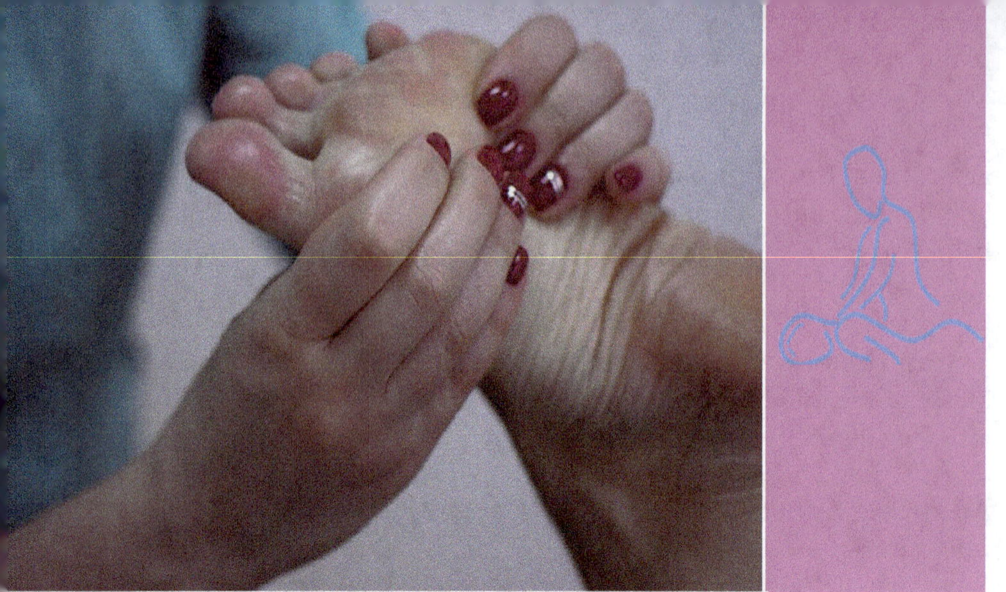

13

REFLEXOLOGY

WHAT YOU'LL LEARN

◊ PHILOSOPHY BEHIND REFLEXOLOGY

◊ REFLEXOLOGY TECHNIQUES

◊ STEP-BY-STEP REFLEXOLOGY

◊ BENEFITS OF REFLEXOLOGY

◊ REFLEXOLOGY MAPS AND KEY REFLEX POINTS

◊ REFLEXOLOGY AND SPECIFIC CONDITIONS

Reflexology is a therapeutic practice rooted in the belief that specific points on the feet, hands, and ears correspond to different organs, systems, and parts of the body. By applying targeted pressure to these areas, reflexology aims to promote relaxation, improve overall health, and support the body's natural healing processes.

In this chapter, we'll explore the principles of reflexology, its benefits, and practical techniques you can incorporate into your daily routine or holistic wellness practice.

The Philosophy Behind Reflexology

Reflexology is based on the idea that the body is interconnected through energy pathways. These pathways, or "zones," run throughout the body and converge at specific points on the feet, hands, and ears. Stimulating these points is thought to balance energy flow, alleviate stress, and encourage the body to heal itself naturally.

While modern reflexology has been influenced by traditional Chinese medicine, similar practices date back to ancient Egypt, India, and other cultures. The concept of mapping the body onto the feet and hands has made reflexology a unique and accessible therapeutic practice.

Reflexology Techniques

1. Thumb Walking:

Using your thumb, apply firm, steady pressure in a walking motion across the reflex points. This technique helps stimulate the corresponding areas of the body.

2. Press and Hold:

Firmly press a specific reflex point for a few seconds before releasing. This method is especially effective for pain relief and relaxation.

3. Circular Motions:

Use your thumb or finger to apply gentle, circular movements on reflex points. This helps improve circulation and energy flow.

4. Alternating Pressure:

Use varying levels of pressure to activate different layers of the reflex point, promoting deeper relaxation and stimulation.

Step-by-Step Reflexology Guide

Below is a step-by-step guide to performing a basic reflexology session on the feet.

Preparation

1. **Create a Relaxing Environment:**

   • Choose a quiet, calm space with soothing music and soft lighting.

   • Ensure the room is warm, as the recipient may be barefoot and partially uncovered.

2. **Gather Supplies:**

   • Comfortable chair or massage table.

   • A towel to support the feet and keep them clean.

   • Optional: Massage oil or lotion, though reflexology is often performed without these.

3. **Understand Reflexology Charts:**

   • Familiarize yourself with a reflexology map to locate pressure points that correspond to specific areas of the body.

4. **Communicate with the Recipient:**

   • Discuss any problem areas, sensitivities, or health conditions.

   • Ensure the recipient is comfortable with touch on their feet or hands.

Step 1: Warm-Up the Feet

1. **Position the Recipient:**

   • Seat them in a comfortable chair or have them lie on a massage table.

   • Support one foot with both hands, ensuring they feel stable and relaxed.

2. **Warm-Up Techniques:**

   • Use light effleurage (stroking) movements to warm up the foot and relax the muscles.

- Rotate the foot gently at the ankle to loosen the joint.

3. Stretch the Toes:

- Gently pull and stretch each toe to release tension.

Step 2: Apply Pressure to the Sole

1. Locate the Reflex Points:

- Refer to a reflexology chart to identify key areas on the sole of the foot that correspond to the recipient's needs.

2. Thumb Walking Technique:

- Use your thumbs to "walk" across the foot in small, incremental steps.

- Press firmly but gently, rolling your thumb from the tip to the pad with each step.

3. Focus on Key Zones:

- **Head and Sinuses:** Work on the tips of the toes.

- **Spine:** Massage the inner edge of the sole, from the heel to the big toe.

- **Digestive System:** Apply pressure to the arch and ball of the foot.

- **Lungs and Chest:** Focus on the area just below the toes on the ball of the foot.

- **Lower Body:** Target the heel and outer edges for the lower back, legs, and hips.

Step 3: Work on Specific Areas

1. Address Tension Points:

- If the recipient mentions specific concerns (e.g., headaches, digestion), spend extra time on the corresponding reflex zones.

2. Apply Circular Pressure:

- Use your thumbs or fingers to apply circular motions to tender spots or knots.

3. Adjust Pressure:

- Be mindful of the recipient's comfort and adjust the intensity of your touch as needed.

Step 4: Focus on the Toes

1. Massage Each Toe Individually:

- Use your thumb and forefinger to gently massage the top, sides, and underside of each toe.

- Pay extra attention to the tips for reflex points connected to the head and sinuses.

2. Squeeze and Roll:

- Squeeze the base of each toe and roll it gently to release tension.

Step 5: Work on the Heel and Ankle

1. Heel Reflex Points:

- Apply firm pressure to the heel, which corresponds to the lower back and pelvic region.

2. Ankle Reflex Points:

- Massage the area around the inner and outer ankle to stimulate reproductive and urinary system reflexes.

3. Circular Motions:

- Use circular movements with your thumb or palm to relax these areas.

Step 6: Repeat on the Other Foot

1. Switch Feet:

- Move to the other foot and repeat all steps, starting with the warm-up.

- Spend equal time on both feet to ensure balance in the treatment.

Step 7: Cool Down and Finish

1. Final Strokes:

- Use light effleurage strokes to relax the feet and signal the end of the session.

2. Stretch and Rotate:

- Gently stretch and rotate each foot to release any remaining

tension.

3. Check-In with the Recipient:

• Ask how they feel and address any lingering tightness or discomfort.

Aftercare Tips

1. Encourage Hydration:

• Suggest drinking water to flush out toxins released during the session.

2. Advise Rest:

• Recommend light activity and rest to allow the body to process the reflexology benefits.

3. Discuss Follow-Up:

• If addressing ongoing issues, suggest regular reflexology sessions for long-term results.

Safety Tips

• **Avoid Reflexology:** If the recipient has open wounds, infections, recent surgeries, or severe circulatory issues.

• **Be Gentle:** Reflexology should never cause pain. Adjust pressure based on feedback.

• **Use Reflexology Charts:** They help ensure you target the correct zones for specific benefits.

Benefits of Reflexology

1. Stress Reduction:

Applying pressure to reflex points can activate the parasympathetic nervous system, promoting deep relaxation and reducing stress-related tension.

.2. Improved Circulation:

Reflexology stimulates blood flow, helping oxygen and nutrients reach tissues and organs more effectively.

3. Enhanced Digestion:

Certain reflex points are associated with the digestive system. Regular reflexology sessions may help alleviate issues like bloating, constipation, and indigestion.

4. Pain Relief:
Reflexology can reduce discomfort from headaches, migraines, back pain, and other chronic conditions by addressing reflex points linked to affected areas.

5. Holistic Balance:
By focusing on the entire body's systems, reflexology promotes balance and harmony, supporting emotional and physical well-being.

Reflexology Maps and Key Reflex Points
Reflexology maps provide a guide to the specific points on the feet, hands, and ears that correspond to different parts of the body.

1. Foot Reflexology Map:

- **Toes:** Head and neck.

- **Ball of the Foot:** Chest, lungs, and upper back.

- **Arch of the Foot:** Digestive organs, including the stomach, **pancreas, and intestines.**

- **Heel:** Pelvic region, lower back, and reproductive organs.

2. Hand Reflexology Map:

- **Fingertips:** Head and neck.

- **Palm:** Vital organs, including the heart, liver, and digestive system.

- **Base of the Hand:** Lower body and spine.

3. Ear Reflexology Map:

- **Lobes:** Head and facial areas.

- **Middle Ear:** Chest and internal organs.

- **Upper Ear:** Lower body and limbs.

Reflexology and Specific Conditions

1. Headaches and Migraines:
Focus on the toes and the tips of the fingers to alleviate head and neck

tension.

2. Digestive Issues:
Massage the arch of the foot or the center of the palm to stimulate the digestive system and relieve discomfort.

3. Anxiety and Stress:
Work on the solar plexus reflex point, located in the middle of the foot, to calm the nervous system.

4. Menstrual Pain:
Target the heel and inner ankle area to ease cramps and support hormonal balance.

Precautions and Best Practices

- **Avoid Overstimulation:** Start with gentle pressure, especially for sensitive or tender reflex points.

- **Medical Conditions:** Consult with a healthcare professional before practicing reflexology if you have conditions like diabetes, circulatory issues, or are pregnant.

- **Stay Hydrated:** Drink plenty of water after a session to help flush out toxins.

- **Consistency is Key:** Regular practice yields the best results for overall health and well-being.

Conclusion
Reflexology is a holistic approach to health that taps into the body's natural healing abilities. By understanding the connections between reflex points and the body's systems, you can harness the power of touch to relieve stress, promote relaxation, and support overall wellness.

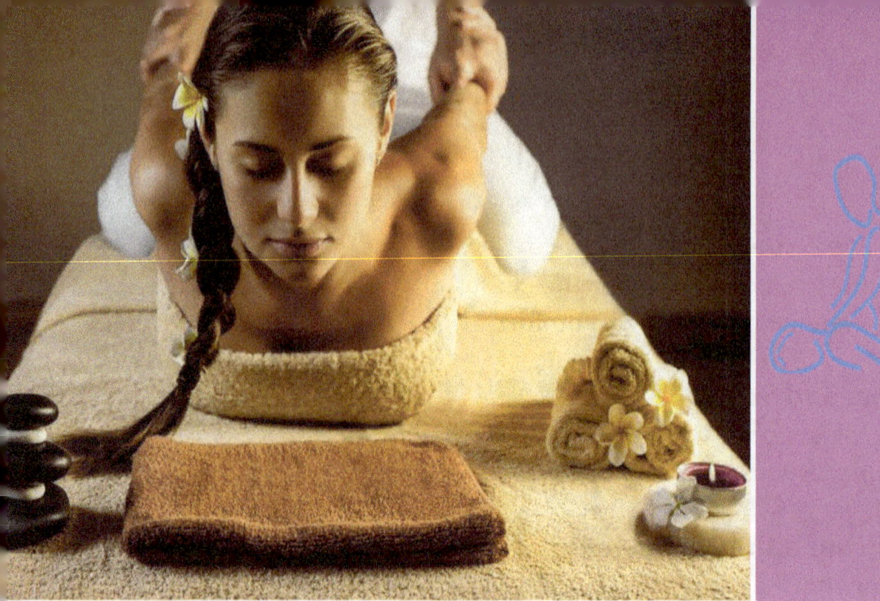

14

THAI MASSAGE

◊ PRINCIPLES OF THAI MASSAGE

◊ TECHNIQUES OF THAI MASSAGE

◊ STEP-BY-STEP THAI MASSAGE

◊ BENEFITS OF THAI MASSAGE

Thai massage, also known as "Nuad Thai," is a traditional healing practice that combines acupressure, stretching, and gentle yoga-like movements to promote balance, flexibility, and energy flow. Rooted in ancient Ayurvedic principles and Thai culture, this dynamic form of bodywork is both invigorating and deeply restorative.

In this chapter, we will explore the history, techniques, benefits, and unique characteristics of Thai massage, as well as how it integrates physical movement with holistic wellness.

The Origins of Thai Massage

Thai massage traces its roots to over 2,500 years ago, with its foundation attributed to Shivago Komarpaj, a physician said to have been a contemporary of the Buddha. Influenced by Indian Ayurvedic medicine and Chinese acupressure, Thai massage evolved as a spiritual and physical healing practice within Thailand's Buddhist temples.

It is often referred to as "Thai yoga massage" because it incorporates rhythmic compressions, deep stretches, and mindful breathing, creating a meditative experience for both the practitioner and the recipient.

Principles of Thai Massage

Thai massage is based on the belief in energy lines, or "Sen," which are similar to meridians in traditional Chinese medicine. These energy pathways are thought to influence the body's physical and emotional well-being. Blockages in the Sen lines can lead to discomfort or illness, and Thai massage aims to release these blockages, restoring balance and vitality.

Unlike other forms of massage, Thai massage is performed on a floor mat, and the recipient remains fully clothed in comfortable, loose-fitting attire. The practitioner uses their hands, elbows, knees, and feet to apply pressure and guide the recipient through assisted stretches.

Techniques of Thai Massage
1. Rhythmic Compression:
Gentle, steady pressure is applied along the Sen lines using the practitioner's hands, palms, elbows, or feet.

2. Assisted Stretching:
Guided stretches, inspired by yoga poses, target specific muscle groups and joints to enhance flexibility.

3. Joint Mobilization:
Movements like gentle rocking and rotation improve joint function and relieve stiffness.

4. Thumb Pressing:
Focused pressure with thumbs is used to release tension in smaller, more sensitive areas.

5. Palming and Footwork:
The practitioner may use their palms or even feet to apply broad, firm pressure across larger muscle groups.

Step-by-Step Thai Massage Guide

Below is a step-by-step guide for performing a basic Thai massage.

Preparation

1. **Set the Environment:**

   - Use a clean, flat mat on the floor.

   - Create a quiet, warm, and peaceful environment with soft lighting.

   - Optional: Play calming music or use aromatherapy for ambiance.

2. **Recipient's Clothing:**

   - Ensure the recipient is wearing loose, comfortable clothing.

3. **Communicate with the Recipient:**

   - Discuss any health concerns, injuries, or problem areas.

   - Explain the process to ensure they feel comfortable and prepared.

4. **Warm-Up Yourself:**

   - Thai massage involves the use of your body weight, so stretch and center yourself before starting to avoid strain.

Step 1: Starting with a Centering Ritual
1. Begin with Breathwork:

- Encourage the recipient to take deep, calming breaths.

- Synchronize your breathing to create a shared sense of relaxation.

2. Palming the Feet:

- Sit at the recipient's feet and gently press the soles with your palms.

- Use slow, rhythmic pressure to establish a connection and introduce touch.

Step 2: Warm-Up the Body with Compression
1. Apply Rhythmic Pressure:

- Use your palms to press down on the recipient's legs, starting from the feet and moving up to the thighs.

- Lean in gently, using your body weight rather than muscular effort.

2. Work Along Energy Lines:

- Focus on "Sen" lines, which are energy pathways in Thai massage.

- Apply pressure with your palms, thumbs, or forearms along the inner and outer legs.

Step 3: Assisted Stretches for the Lower Body
1. Hamstring Stretch:

- Raise one leg while the recipient lies flat on their back.

- Press the leg toward their torso, keeping the knee straight, and hold for a few breaths.

2. Hip Opener Stretch:

- Bend one knee and bring it toward the opposite shoulder.

- Use your hands to gently guide the movement, opening up the hip joint.

3. Butterfly Stretch:

- With the recipient's soles together and knees bent, gently press down on their knees to stretch the inner thighs.

Step 4: Work on the Upper Body

1. Shoulder and Chest Compression:

- Move to the head of the mat and press your palms on the recipient's shoulders.

- Use steady, downward pressure to release tension.

2. Seated Upper Body Stretch:

- Help the recipient sit upright with their legs crossed.

- Stand behind them and gently pull their arms backward, opening the chest and stretching the shoulders.

3. Twist Stretch:

- Guide the recipient into a seated twist by placing one hand on their opposite knee and the other hand on the floor behind them.

- Support the movement to ensure a deep but comfortable stretch.

Step 5: Side-Lying Position

1. Back Compression:

- With the recipient lying on their side, use your palms to press along their back, focusing on the shoulder blades and lower back.

2. Leg Stretch:

- Hold the top leg at the knee and ankle, stretching it gently upward and outward.

3. Spinal Twist:

- Guide the recipient into a side-lying spinal twist by pulling the top leg across their body while pressing their shoulder in the opposite direction.

Step 6: Focus on the Back

1. Palm and Thumb Pressure:

- Have the recipient lie on their stomach. Use your palms and thumbs to press along the spine and shoulders.

2. **Cat Stretch:**

   • Stand over the recipient and gently lift their arms backward while they lie on their stomach, creating a deep back stretch.

2. **Kneeling Back Stretch:**

   • Ask the recipient to kneel while you kneel behind them. Place your hands on their shoulders and gently press downward to stretch the spine.

Step 7: End with Relaxation

1. **Face and Scalp Massage:**

   • Have the recipient lie on their back. Use your fingertips to massage their temples, forehead, and scalp with gentle, circular motions.

2. **Palm and Foot Pressure:**

   • Finish with light pressure on the recipient's palms and soles to ground their energy.

3. **Closing Gesture:**

   • Press your hands together in a prayer position, thanking the recipient for allowing you to share the session.

Aftercare Tips

1. **Hydration:**

   • Encourage the recipient to drink water to flush out toxins and rehydrate.

2. **Rest:**

   • Suggest a period of relaxation after the session to allow the body to absorb the benefits.

3. **Stretching:**

   • Recommend gentle stretching to maintain the flexibility gained during the massage.

Safety Tips

   • **Adjust Pressure:** Always tailor the pressure to the recipient's comfort level.

   • **Avoid Overstretching:** Be mindful of the recipient's limits during assisted stretches.

- **Contraindications:** Avoid Thai massage if the recipient has injuries, recent surgeries, or conditions such as osteoporosis or severe arthritis.

Benefits of Thai Massage

1. Enhances Flexibility and Range of Motion:
Stretching movements gently open up the body, improving flexibility and reducing stiffness.

2. Relieves Muscle Tension and Pain:
Targeted pressure and stretches release knots and tension, particularly in the back, shoulders, and legs.

3. Boosts Circulation and Energy Flow:
By stimulating the Sen lines, Thai massage encourages better blood and lymph circulation, leading to increased energy levels.

4. Reduces Stress and Promotes Relaxation:
The combination of rhythmic movements and mindful breathing calms the mind and relaxes the nervous system.

5. Improves Posture and Alignment:
Deep stretches and joint mobilization help correct imbalances, promoting better posture.

6. Supports Emotional Well-Being:
Thai massage's meditative nature fosters a sense of connection, grounding, and inner peace.

Precautions and Considerations

- **Medical Conditions:** Consult with a healthcare provider before receiving Thai massage if you have conditions such as joint issues, chronic pain, or pregnancy.

- **Communicate Needs:** Inform your therapist about any discomfort or sensitive areas during the session.

- **Proper Training:** If practicing Thai massage on others, seek formal training to ensure safety and effectiveness.

Conclusion

Thai massage is much more than a physical therapy—it is a harmonious blend of movement, mindfulness, and healing. Rooted in ancient traditions, it offers a pathway to relaxation, flexibility, and balance for the body and mind.

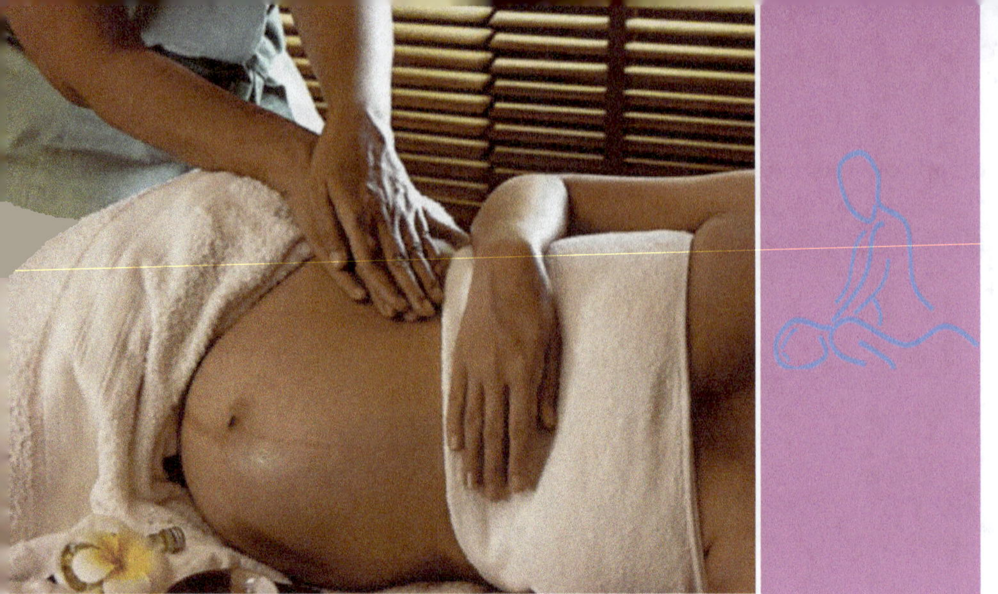

15

PRENATAL MASSAGE

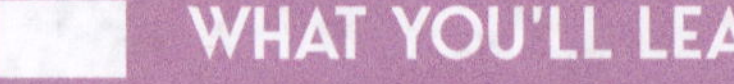

WHAT YOU'LL LEARN

◊ WHAT IS PRENATAL MASSAGE?

◊ TECHNIQUES USED IN PRENATAL MASSAGE

◊ STEP-BY-STEP PRENATAL MASSAGE

◊ BENEFITS OF PRENATAL MASSAGE

◊ ADDRESSING COMMON PREGNANACY

DISCOMFORTS

Prenatal massage is a specialized form of therapy designed to support and nurture women during pregnancy. It addresses the unique physical and emotional changes that occur during this transformative time, offering relief from discomfort, promoting relaxation, and fostering a deeper connection between mother and baby.

In this chapter, we'll explore the benefits of prenatal massage, techniques, safety considerations, and how this gentle therapy can enhance well-being throughout pregnancy.

What is Prenatal Massage?

Prenatal massage is tailored to the needs of expectant mothers at every stage of pregnancy. It combines techniques like gentle kneading, light stroking, and positional adjustments to address pregnancy-related discomforts while ensuring the safety and comfort of both mother and baby.

This type of massage is performed with the mother lying on her side or supported by specially designed cushions to accommodate her growing belly.

Techniques Used in Prenatal Massage

1. Swedish Massage Techniques:
Gentle, flowing strokes are used to promote relaxation, reduce muscle tension, and improve circulation.

2. Light Stretching:
Careful stretches can alleviate tension in the hips and lower back, areas that often bear the brunt of pregnancy-related discomfort.

3. Gentle Pressure Points:
Avoiding contraindicated points, light pressure can relieve tension and promote relaxation in safe areas like the shoulders and feet.

4. Side-Lying Positioning:
This position ensures comfort and safety, with support from pillows or bolsters to relieve pressure on the abdomen and lower back.

Step-by-Step Prenatal Massage Guide

Prenatal massage is designed to support the unique needs of pregnant individuals, promoting relaxation, reducing stress, and alleviating common discomforts like back pain and swelling. Always consult the client's healthcare provider before offering a prenatal massage and tailor your approach based on the pregnancy stage and the client's comfort.

Preparation

1. **Ensure a Safe Environment:**

   • Choose a warm, quiet room with calming music and soft lighting.

   • Ensure the client feels secure and comfortable.

2. **Use Proper Equipment:**

   • A firm but comfortable massage table.

   • Pillows, bolsters, or specialized pregnancy cushions to support side-lying positions.

3. **Choose Safe Products:**

   • Use unscented or pregnancy-safe oils and lotions to avoid triggering sensitivities.

4. **Communicate with the Client:**

   • Discuss any pregnancy-related discomfort, medical conditions, or areas to avoid.

   • Confirm they are comfortable with touch and the session plan.

Step 1: Position the Client Safely

1. **Side-Lying Position:**

   • Most prenatal massages are performed in a side-lying position for safety and comfort.

   • Use pillows to support the head, belly, and between the knees.

2. **Alternative Positions:**

   • Semi-reclined for upper body work or seated in a supportive chair for short sessions.

   • Avoid prone (lying on the stomach) or supine (lying flat on the back after the first trimester).

Step 2: Start with the Back

1. Side-Lying Back Massage:

- Begin with gentle effleurage (long, sweeping strokes) along the back to promote relaxation.

- Use your palms to apply light to medium pressure, working from the lower back to the shoulders.

2. Target Tension Points:

- Focus on the upper back, shoulders, and lower back, where tension commonly builds.

- Avoid deep pressure on the lower back and sacral area, especially during later trimesters.

3. Soothing Strokes:

- Use circular motions with your hands or fingertips to release tightness along the spine and shoulder blades.

Step 3: Address the Legs and Feet

1. Gentle Compression on the Legs:

- Start at the upper thighs and work downward toward the feet with light pressure to promote circulation.

2. Avoid Certain Areas:

- Do not apply deep pressure to the inner thighs, calves, or ankles due to the risk of triggering sensitive points.

3. Foot Massage:

- Use your thumbs to apply gentle pressure to the soles, avoiding acupressure points linked to labor induction.

- Massage the arches and heels to relieve soreness and swelling.

Step 4: Focus on the Arms and Hands

1. Effleurage on the Arms:

- Use long, soothing strokes from the shoulders to the hands.

2. Hand Massage:

- Massage each finger, palm, and wrist using circular motions.

- This can help reduce tension caused by fluid retention.

Step 5: Alleviate Neck and Shoulder Tension
  1. **Gentle Shoulder Strokes:**

   • Massage the tops of the shoulders with light to medium pressure, avoiding any discomfort.

  2. **Neck Massage:**

   • Use your fingertips to apply gentle circular motions along the neck, avoiding direct pressure on the spine.

Step 6: Optional Belly Massage (If Requested)
  1. **Communicate First:**

   • Offer a belly massage only if the client is comfortable with it.

   • Use light, soothing strokes to reduce tension in the abdominal area.

  2. **Technique:**

   • Gently apply oil or lotion and use slow, circular motions to relax the muscles.

   • Avoid applying any pressure directly to the belly.

Step 7: Closing the Massage
  1. **Soothing Strokes:**

   • End with gentle, rhythmic strokes on the back, arms, or legs to leave the client feeling relaxed and grounded.

  2. **Transition Slowly:**

   • Help the client sit up gradually, as sudden movements may cause dizziness.

  3. **Check-In:**

   • Ask how they feel and if there are any lingering areas of discomfort.

Aftercare Tips
  1. **Hydration:**

   • Encourage the client to drink water to stay hydrated and help flush out toxins.

  2. **Rest:**

   • Suggest taking time to relax after the massage to fully enjoy its benefits.

3. Follow-Up:

- Discuss regular sessions to address ongoing discomforts and promote relaxation throughout pregnancy.

Important Considerations

1. Avoid Contraindicated Areas:

- Do not apply pressure to sensitive areas like the inner thighs, ankles, or certain acupressure points.

2. Be Mindful of Trimester:

- Tailor the session to the stage of pregnancy. For example:

    - **First trimester:** Focus on relaxation and avoid deep pressure.

    - **Second trimester:** Address growing discomforts, such as back pain or swelling.

    - **Third trimester:** Prioritize comfort and light pressure.

3. Seek Professional Guidance:

- If unsure, consult a certified prenatal massage therapist or healthcare provider.

Benefits of Prenatal Massage

1. Relieves Physical Discomfort:

- Alleviates back pain, hip discomfort, and sciatica caused by the added weight and shifting posture during pregnancy.

- Reduces swelling in the hands, feet, and legs by improving circulation and lymphatic flow.

2. Reduces Stress and Anxiety:

- Promotes relaxation and emotional well-being by reducing cortisol levels and boosting serotonin production.

3. Improves Sleep Quality:

- Relaxes tense muscles and calms the nervous system, helping mothers sleep better.

4. Supports Circulation:

- Enhances blood flow, ensuring oxygen and nutrients reach the baby more effectively.

5. Eases Hormonal Changes:

- Can help balance mood swings and alleviate symptoms of anxiety or depression.

6. Prepares for Labor:

- Improves flexibility and muscle tone in preparation for childbirth.

Addressing Common Pregnancy Discomforts
1. Back Pain:

- Gentle kneading and pressure on the lower back can relieve tension caused by changes in posture and weight distribution.

2. Swelling (Edema):

- Massage techniques that stimulate lymphatic drainage help reduce fluid retention in the extremities.

3. Leg Cramps:

- Light strokes and stretches in the calves can alleviate cramps and improve circulation.

4. Hip Pain:

- Focused work around the hips and pelvis can ease discomfort as ligaments loosen in preparation for childbirth.

Creating a Relaxing Prenatal Massage Experience
1. Comfortable Environment:

- Use soft lighting, soothing music, and warm blankets to create a calming atmosphere.

2. Supportive Positioning:

- Ensure the mother feels secure and comfortable with cushions and bolsters.

3. Incorporate Aromatherapy:

- Use pregnancy-safe essential oils, such as lavender or chamomile, to enhance relaxation (avoid contraindicated oils).

4. Encourage Mindful Breathing:

- Integrate deep breathing exercises to deepen relaxation and promote a sense of calm.

Prenatal Massage and Emotional Connection

Prenatal massage isn't just about physical relief—it can also foster a stronger bond between mother and baby. The relaxation and mindfulness encouraged during sessions create a space for expectant mothers to connect with their baby, focusing on their shared journey.

For partners, learning simple prenatal massage techniques can also be a meaningful way to support and bond with the mother-to-be, deepening emotional intimacy during this special time.

Postnatal Benefits

While the focus of this chapter is on pregnancy, it's worth noting that massage therapy continues to be beneficial after childbirth. Postnatal massage can help with recovery, reducing muscle tension, and addressing postpartum emotional changes.

Conclusion

Prenatal massage is a gentle, nurturing therapy that supports expectant mothers through the physical and emotional changes of pregnancy. With its ability to alleviate discomfort, reduce stress, and prepare the body for childbirth, prenatal massage is a valuable tool for promoting overall well-being during this transformative journey.

Whether it's through regular professional sessions or simple at-home techniques shared with a partner, prenatal massage offers a soothing way to celebrate and care for the incredible process of bringing new life into the world.

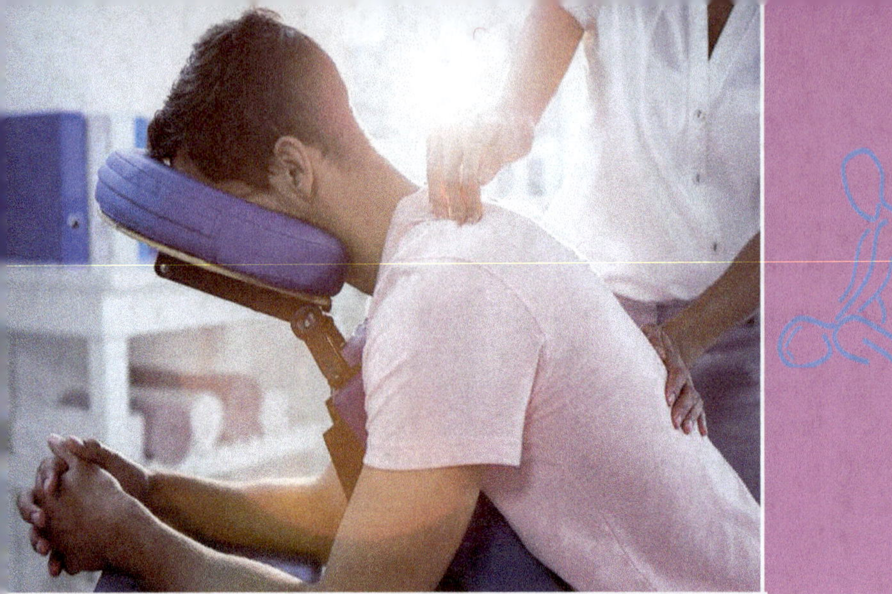

16

CHAIR MASSAGE

WHAT YOU'LL LEARN

◊ WHAT IS CHAIR MASSAGE?

◊ TECHNIQUES USED IN CHAIR MASSAGE

◊ STEP-BY-STEP CHAIR MASSAGE

◊ BENEFITS OF CHAIR MASSAGE

◊ WHERE CHAIR MASSAGE IS COMMONLY

OFFERED

Chair massage is a quick, accessible form of therapy designed to relieve tension and promote relaxation without requiring a traditional massage table. This type of massage is often performed in a seated position using a specially designed chair that provides ergonomic support for the head, arms, and back.

Whether at the office, a wellness event, or even a shopping mall, chair massage offers a convenient way to experience the benefits of massage therapy in as little as 10 to 30 minutes.

What is Chair Massage?

Chair massage focuses primarily on the upper body, including the back, shoulders, neck, arms, and head. Clients remain fully clothed, making it a versatile and comfortable option for those new to massage or seeking quick relief from tension.

The massage is performed using a combination of techniques, such as kneading, compression, and rhythmic strokes, tailored to the individual's needs.

Techniques Used in Chair Massage

1. Effleurage (Gliding Strokes):
Gentle, sweeping strokes are used to warm up the muscles and promote relaxation.

2. Petrissage (Kneading):
Kneading techniques target tight muscles, especially in the shoulders and upper back.

3. Compression:
Applying gentle pressure to muscle groups helps improve circulation and release tension.

4. Percussion (Tapotement):
Rhythmic tapping motions can invigorate the body and stimulate the muscles.

5. Friction:
Small, circular motions help break up knots and relieve localized tension.

Step-by-Step Chair Massage Guide

Below is a step-by-step guide for giving a professional chair massage.

Preparation

1. Set Up the Massage Chair:

- Adjust the chair height and angle to suit the recipient's body size and comfort.

- Ensure the chair is stable and secure.

2. Create a Comfortable Environment:

- Choose a quiet space with minimal distractions.

- Offer optional soothing music or aromatherapy for relaxation.

3. Communicate with the Recipient:

- Ask about any areas of tension, pain, or medical conditions.

- Explain the process, ensuring they're comfortable with the techniques you'll use.

4. Position the Recipient:

- Ask them to sit facing the chair with their chest resting on the chest pad, arms supported on the armrest, and face comfortably in the face cradle.

- Adjust the settings to maintain a neutral spine and relaxed posture.

Step 1: Start with the Back

1. Warm-Up with Effleurage:

- Use your palms to perform long, sweeping strokes along the back to warm up the muscles.

- Begin at the shoulders and move down to the lower back, applying moderate pressure.

2. Apply Compression:

- Use your palms or fists to gently compress the muscles along the back, focusing on the shoulder blades and spine.

- Avoid pressing directly on the spine.

3. Circular Motions:

- Use your thumbs or fingers to make circular motions along the muscles on either side of the spine.

- Work on tight areas gently but firmly.

Step 2: Focus on the Shoulders
1. Kneading:

- Use your fingers and thumbs to knead the shoulder muscles, similar to kneading dough.

- Apply more pressure to areas of tension, but ensure the recipient is comfortable.

2. Pinching:

- Lightly pinch and lift the top of the shoulders to release tension.

- Use rhythmic motions for a relaxing effect.

3. Rolling:

- Roll the shoulder muscles under your palms or fingers to increase circulation and release stiffness.

Step 3: Address the Neck
1. Thumb Pressure:

- Use your thumbs to apply gentle pressure along the neck, moving from the base of the skull down to the shoulders.

2. Circular Motions:

- Massage the neck muscles in small, circular motions, focusing on areas of stiffness.

3. Stretching:

- Gently tilt the recipient's head side-to-side to stretch the neck muscles.

- Always move slowly and within the recipient's comfort range.

Step 4: Work on the Arms and Hands
1. Arm Massage:

- Use long, sweeping strokes to massage the upper arms, moving down toward the forearms.

- Apply moderate pressure and use kneading motions to relieve muscle tension.

2. Hand Massage:

- Massage the palms with your thumbs in circular motions.

- Gently stretch each finger, pulling lightly from the base to the tip.

3. Wrist Relaxation:

- Use your fingers to gently rotate the wrists in both directions to ease stiffness.

Step 5: Focus on the Head and Scalp

1. Scalp Massage:

- Use your fingertips to make small circular motions across the scalp.

- Apply gentle pressure, moving from the forehead to the back of the head.

2. Temples and Jawline:

- Massage the temples in circular motions to relieve stress.

- Apply light pressure along the jawline to release tension from clenching.

Step 6: Finish with Relaxation

1. Gentle Back Strokes:

- Perform light, soothing strokes across the back to signal the end of the session.

2. Grounding Touch:

- Place your hands lightly on the recipient's shoulders for a few seconds to create a grounding effect.

3. Encourage Deep Breathing:

- Invite the recipient to take a few deep breaths before transitioning out of the chair.

Aftercare Tips

1. Hydration:

- Suggest the recipient drink water to rehydrate and support toxin release.

2. **Stretching:**

- Recommend light stretches for the neck, shoulders, and back to maintain the benefits of the massage.

3. **Feedback:**

- Ask for feedback to understand what techniques were most effective and areas to focus on in the future.

Safety Considerations

- **Avoid High-Risk Areas:** Do not apply pressure to the spine, abdomen, or areas of injury.

- **Tailor Pressure:** Adjust pressure based on the recipient's comfort level.

- **Medical Conditions:** Avoid chair massage if the recipient has certain medical issues (e.g., recent surgeries, fractures, or severe inflammation).

Benefits of Chair Massage

1. Reduces Stress:

Chair massage is highly effective at reducing stress and anxiety, promoting a sense of calm even during a busy day.

2. Relieves Muscle Tension:

Focused work on common problem areas, such as the neck and shoulders, helps alleviate muscle tightness caused by poor posture or repetitive activities.

3. Boosts Energy and Focus:

A brief chair massage can improve circulation and stimulate the nervous system, leaving you feeling recharged and alert.

4. Improves Workplace Productivity:

Offering chair massages in the office has been shown to enhance employee morale, reduce absenteeism, and improve overall productivity.

5. Increases Accessibility:

Chair massage is an excellent option for people who may feel uncomfortable with traditional table massage or have time constraints.

Where Chair Massage is Commonly Offered

1. Corporate Wellness Programs:
Many companies include chair massage as part of their wellness initiatives to help employees manage stress.

2. Public Events and Trade Shows:
Chair massage is a popular feature at events, offering attendees a moment to relax and recharge.

3. Gyms and Fitness Centers:
Post-workout chair massages help relieve muscle soreness and promote recovery.

4. Shopping Malls and Airports:
Chair massage kiosks provide a convenient option for relaxation during errands or long layovers.

5. Private Parties or Gatherings:
Hiring a chair massage therapist can add a unique, relaxing element to social events.

Chair Massage for Stress Relief

Chair massage is particularly effective at targeting stress-related tension. Daily activities, such as sitting at a desk, driving, or using digital devices, often result in tightness in the shoulders, neck, and upper back. By focusing on these areas, chair massage provides quick relief, helping you return to your day feeling refreshed and reenergized.

Conclusion

Chair massage offers a quick, effective way to relax, relieve tension, and improve overall well-being. Its accessibility and convenience make it an excellent option for anyone looking to experience the benefits of massage therapy without the need for a lengthy session or special preparations.

Whether enjoyed at work, at an event, or in the comfort of your own home, chair massage is a wonderful reminder that even a few minutes of focused care can make a world of difference for your body and mind.

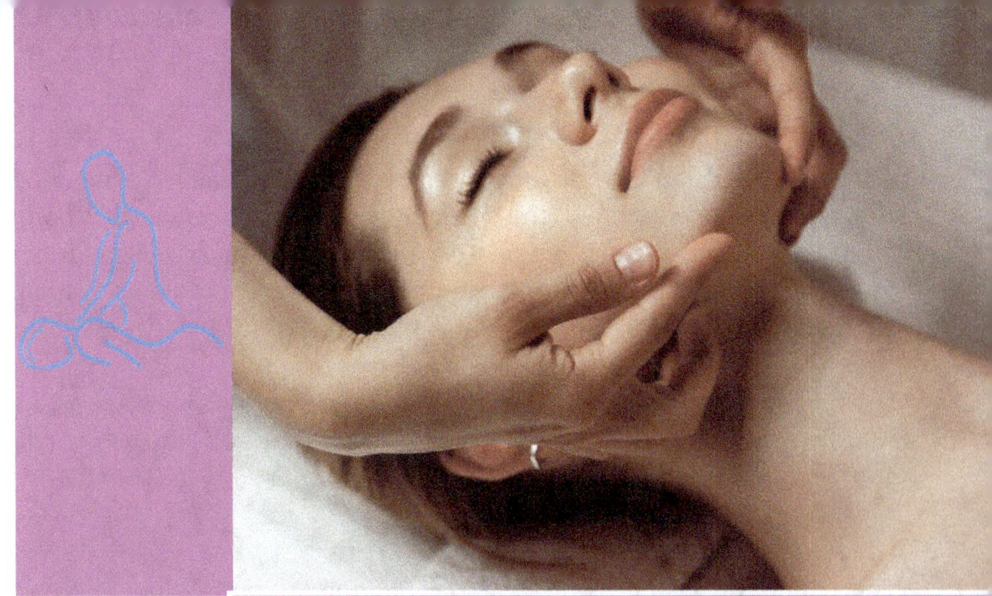

17

LYMPHATIC DRAINAGE MASSAGE

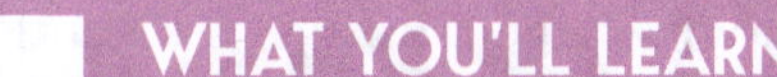

WHAT YOU'LL LEARN

◊ WHAT IS LYMPHATIC DRAINAGE MASSAGE?

◊ TECHNIQUES USED IN LYMPHATIC DRAINAGE MASSAGE

◊ STEP-BY-STEP LYMPHATIC DRAINAGE MASSAGE

◊ BENEFITS OF LYMPHATIC DRAINAGE MASSAGE

Lymphatic drainage massage is a gentle and specialized technique designed to stimulate the lymphatic system, helping the body naturally remove toxins and waste. This form of massage not only promotes overall health but also supports recovery, reduces swelling, and enhances immunity.

In this chapter, we'll explore what lymphatic drainage massage is, its benefits, techniques, and how it can be incorporated into a holistic approach to wellness.

Understanding the Lymphatic System

The lymphatic system is an essential part of the body's immune and circulatory systems. It consists of lymph nodes, vessels, and fluid (lymph), which work together to:

- Remove toxins and waste from tissues.

- Transport white blood cells to fight infection.

- Maintain fluid balance in the body.

Unlike the circulatory system, the lymphatic system doesn't have a pump like the heart. It relies on muscle movements, breathing, and manual stimulation, such as lymphatic drainage massage, to keep the fluid flowing.

What is Lymphatic Drainage Massage?

Lymphatic drainage massage is a gentle, rhythmic massage technique that follows the natural pathways of the lymphatic system. The goal is to encourage the movement of lymph, helping the body detoxify and reduce swelling.

This type of massage is often used:

- After surgery to reduce post-operative swelling.

- To support conditions like lymphedema.

- As part of a general wellness routine to enhance detoxification.

Techniques Used in Lymphatic Drainage Massage

1. Gentle Strokes:

Light, repetitive movements are used to encourage the flow of lymph.

Unlike traditional massage, there's no deep pressure involved.

2. Pumping Motions:
Specific areas, like the neck and armpits, are targeted with soft, pumping motions to stimulate lymph nodes.

3. Directional Movements:
Strokes follow the natural flow of the lymphatic system, moving fluid toward the lymph nodes.

4. Circular Motions:
Small, circular motions are applied around areas prone to congestion, such as the neck and face.

Step-by-Step Lymphatic Drainage Massage Guide
Below is a step-by-step guide to performing lymphatic drainage massage.
Preparation
1. **Create a Relaxing Environment:**

   - Choose a calm and quiet space, free from distractions.

   - Dim the lights and play soothing music to promote relaxation.

2. **Consult the Client:**

   - Ask the client if they have any medical conditions, allergies, or contraindications such as active infections, heart problems, or blood clotting disorders.

   - Discuss any areas of tension or swelling that need to be addressed.

3. **Choose Appropriate Oils or Lotions:**

   - Use light, non-greasy oils or lotions that allow for smooth movements without creating friction. Essential oils like lavender, chamomile, or geranium may also be used to enhance relaxation.

4. **Position the Client:**

   - Have the client lie comfortably on a massage table, with a cushion or pillow for added support, especially under the knees for comfort.

   - If working on the face, ensure the client is comfortably

positioned with their face down or slightly turned.

Step 1: Start with Breathing Techniques

1. Guide Deep Breathing:

- Encourage the client to take slow, deep breaths in through the nose and out through the mouth.

- Deep breathing helps to activate the lymphatic system and promotes relaxation, so take a few minutes to focus on this before starting the massage.

Step 2: Perform the Initial Light Strokes

1. Neck Strokes (Cervical Lymph Nodes):

- Begin by gently massaging the sides of the neck using light strokes towards the collarbones, where lymph nodes are concentrated.

- Use your fingertips or palms to make gentle, sweeping strokes, moving in the direction of lymph flow. Repeat 5–10 times on both sides.

2. Clavicle Area:

- Apply light pressure to the clavicle (collarbone) area, using circular motions to stimulate the lymph nodes located there.

- This helps to clear the area for the rest of the lymphatic drainage massage.

Step 3: Perform Gentle Strokes on the Limbs

1. Arms and Hands:

- Start at the wrists or hands and use light, gentle strokes towards the shoulder, always moving in the direction of the heart (towards the lymphatic drainage points).

- Use a combination of effleurage (long, smooth strokes) and light pumping motions to stimulate lymph flow.

- Be sure to use light pressure to avoid compressing the lymphatic vessels.

2. Legs and Feet:

- Start from the ankles or feet and work upwards towards the groin, where lymphatic fluid drains.

•   Use your palms or fingers to perform soft, circular motions along the legs, then move up with smooth, long strokes.

•   Repeat on both legs, always moving toward the lymphatic drainage points.

Step 4: Focus on the Abdomen
  1. Gentle Circular Motions on the Stomach:

•   Use light, circular motions with your palms around the abdomen, following the natural flow of the lymphatic system.

•   Focus on the area above the belly button, moving in a clockwise direction to mimic the direction of lymphatic flow.

•   Apply light pressure, ensuring the massage is soothing and relaxing.

Step 5: Drain the Upper Body and Head
  1. Shoulders:

•   Use gentle strokes to work on the shoulder area. Place your hands on the upper back and slowly massage in circular movements, moving toward the lymphatic drainage points under the armpits and down towards the collarbones.

  2. Face and Neck (Optional):

•   If the client is comfortable, perform gentle lymphatic drainage on the face. Use your fingertips to lightly stroke the jawline, cheeks, and forehead.

•   Follow the lymphatic pathways towards the ears and down to the neck. Be extremely gentle around the delicate facial area.

•   You can use very light pressure to avoid any discomfort.

Step 6: Complete the Massage with Final Drainage Techniques
  1. Revisit the Neck and Clavicle Area:

•   Return to the neck and clavicle area to stimulate the final clearing of the lymphatic pathways.

•   Use gentle, rhythmic strokes towards the collarbone to ensure all the lymph fluid is properly drained.

2.**Final Gentle Strokes:**

- Use soft, calming strokes on the entire body to finish the session. Focus on areas that may have felt tense or swollen.

- Allow a few minutes of light effleurage strokes along the back, arms, and legs to soothe and calm the client.

Aftercare Tips

1. Hydration:

- Encourage the client to drink plenty of water after the massage to help flush out any toxins released during the session.

2. Rest and Relaxation:

- Recommend that the client rests for at least an hour after the session to allow the lymphatic system to continue its natural process.

3. Avoid Tight Clothing:

- Advise wearing loose-fitting clothing after the massage to avoid restricting lymphatic flow.

4. Regular Sessions:

- Suggest regular lymphatic drainage massage for continued benefits, particularly for individuals with edema or fluid retention.

Important Considerations

- **Light Pressure:** Always apply light, gentle pressure as the lymphatic system operates at a low pressure, and too much force can impede fluid flow.

- **Contraindications:** Lymphatic drainage massage should not be performed on individuals with active infections, cancer, blood clotting disorders, or acute inflammation. Always check for contraindications before starting.

- **Sensitivity:** Some clients may be sensitive to touch or pressure, so ensure to adapt your pressure based on their comfort level.

Benefits of Lymphatic Drainage Massage

1. Reduces Swelling and Fluid Retention:

By improving lymph flow, the massage helps reduce edema and puffiness, especially in areas like the legs, arms, and face.

2. Enhances Immune Function:
Stimulating the lymphatic system supports the removal of toxins and boosts the body's natural defense mechanisms.

3. Improves Skin Health:
Lymphatic drainage promotes circulation and detoxification, leading to clearer, healthier-looking skin.

4. Aids in Recovery:
After surgery or injury, this massage helps speed up healing by reducing swelling and supporting tissue repair.

5. Promotes Relaxation:
The slow, gentle techniques calm the nervous system, providing stress relief and a sense of well-being.

Who Can Benefit from Lymphatic Drainage Massage?

1. Post-Surgical Patients:
This massage is often recommended after cosmetic or medical surgeries to reduce swelling and speed up recovery.

2. Individuals with Lymphedema:
People with conditions affecting lymphatic flow can benefit from regular sessions to manage symptoms.

3. Those Experiencing Swelling or Puffiness:
Fluid retention from travel, hormonal changes, or other factors can be alleviated.

4. Wellness Enthusiasts:
Many include lymphatic drainage in their routine for its detoxifying and relaxing effects.

Facial Lymphatic Drainage Massage

Facial lymphatic drainage massage has gained popularity for its beauty benefits. It helps reduce puffiness, improve circulation, and give the skin a radiant glow.

Key techniques include:

- **Light sweeps along the jawline:** To reduce puffiness and enhance definition.

- **Circular motions around the eyes:** To alleviate dark circles and swelling.

- **Strokes down the neck:** To promote drainage toward the lymph nodes.

When to Avoid Lymphatic Drainage Massage

While lymphatic drainage massage is generally safe, it may not be suitable for everyone. Consult a healthcare provider before undergoing this treatment if you have:

- Active infections or inflammation.

- Congestive heart failure.

- Blood clots or thrombosis.

- Severe kidney issues.

Conclusion

Lymphatic drainage massage is a gentle yet powerful way to support your body's natural detox processes and promote overall health. Whether you're recovering from surgery, managing swelling, or simply seeking relaxation, this massage technique offers a wealth of benefits.

By understanding the principles and techniques of lymphatic drainage, you can incorporate this therapy into your wellness routine, enhancing your body's ability to heal and thrive.

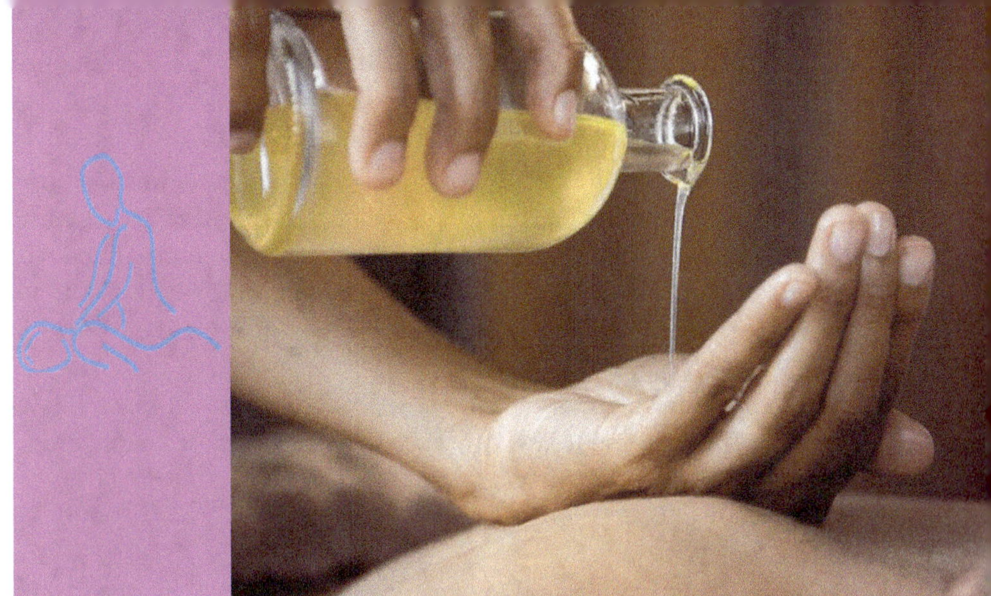

18

ABHYANGA OIL MASSAGE

WHAT YOU'LL LEARN

◊ WHAT IS ABHYANGA OIL MASSAGE?

◊ TECHNIQUES OF ABHYANGA OIL MASSAGE

◊ STEP-BY-STEP ABHYANGA OIL MASSAGE

◊ BENEFITS OF ABHYANGA OIL MASSAGE

◊ TYPES OF OILS USED IN ABHYANGA

Abhyanga is an ancient Ayurvedic practice that involves the application of warm herbal oils to the body, followed by a gentle, rhythmic massage. This form of massage has been practiced for thousands of years in India and is central to Ayurvedic healing, known for its detoxifying, rejuvenating, and stress-relieving benefits.

In this chapter, we'll explore the benefits of Abhyanga oil massage, its techniques, the oils used, and how it can help promote balance and wellness in your life.

What is Abhyanga?

Abhyanga is a traditional Ayurvedic practice that involves self-massage (or receiving a massage) using warm, medicinal oils that are chosen based on the individual's dosha, or constitution, and current health condition.

According to Ayurveda, the body is composed of three primary energies, or doshas: Vata, Pitta, and Kapha. Each person has a unique balance of these energies, which determines their physical, emotional, and mental makeup.

The goal of Abhyanga is to restore balance and harmony by addressing imbalances in these energies, which can lead to various health issues if left unchecked. The massage is performed using oils that are specifically selected for their therapeutic qualities and tailored to the individual's needs.

Techniques of Abhyanga Oil Massage

Abhyanga oil massage is performed using long, flowing strokes, gentle kneading, and circular motions. The technique used will depend on the individual's needs and the areas of the body being addressed.

1. Long, Stoking Movements

Starting from the extremities (hands, feet), the therapist applies gentle, long strokes to move the oil towards the heart. This technique helps improve circulation and lymphatic drainage.

2. Circular Movements on Joints

The therapist uses circular motions over the joints (elbows, knees, and shoulders) to increase mobility and relieve stiffness.

3. Kneading and Tapping
Gentle kneading and tapping techniques help to release muscle tension, especially in areas of the body prone to tightness, such as the neck and back.

4. Abdominal Massage
Circular strokes on the abdomen are designed to stimulate digestion and improve the function of the digestive system, promoting balance in the stomach and intestines.

Step-by-Step Abhyanga Oil Massage Guide
Abhyanga is an integral part of Ayurvedic health and wellness routines, promoting relaxation, vitality, and overall well-being.
Below is a step-by-step guide for performing an Abhyanga oil massage.
Preparation
1. **Choose the Right Oil:**

   - Select an oil based on the client's dosha (Vata, Pitta, or Kapha) or specific needs.

      - For Vata: Sesame oil, which is grounding and warming.

      - For Pitta: Coconut oil or sunflower oil, which are cooling and soothing.

      - For Kapha: Mustard oil or a blend with essential oils that stimulate circulation.

2. **Warm the Oil:**

   - Warm the oil to a comfortable temperature, around 38-40 degrees (100-104 Fahrenheit). You can use a double boiler or a small heating pad to ensure the oil is warm but not scalding.

3. **Prepare the Space:**

   - Create a calming, peaceful environment with dim lights and soft music.

   - Use a massage table or a comfortable surface where the client can lie down, ensuring privacy and warmth.

• Have towels and linens ready to cover the client during the massage.

4. **Consult the Client:**

   • Ask the client about any specific areas of tension or discomfort.

   • Ensure the client does not have any contraindications for oil massage, such as skin sensitivities or allergies.

Step 1: Begin with a Relaxing Breathing Exercise

1. **Guide Deep Breathing:**

   • Invite the client to take slow, deep breaths in through the nose and out through the mouth.

   • This encourages relaxation, calms the nervous system, and prepares the body for the massage.

Step 2: Start with the Head and Face

1. **Massage the Scalp:**

   • Pour a small amount of warm oil onto your palms and gently rub your hands together.

   • Begin massaging the scalp using your fingertips in circular motions, starting at the crown of the head.

   • Move in small, gentle circles, applying pressure to release tension. This helps stimulate the scalp, promoting relaxation and nourishment.

2. **Facial Massage:**

   • Apply a few drops of oil to your fingertips and begin massaging the face in upward circular strokes.

   • Focus on areas like the temples, forehead, and jaw. Use gentle pressure around the eyes and cheeks.

   • The face can be massaged using light strokes to promote relaxation and improve circulation.

Step 3: Massage the Upper Body

1. **Shoulders and Neck:**

   • Pour a bit more oil onto your palms and begin by applying long, gentle strokes down the shoulders and neck.

- Use circular motions at the base of the neck and the tops of the shoulders to release tension.

- Alternate between long strokes and kneading to work out knots and tight muscles.

2. Arms:

- Massage the arms using long, sweeping strokes from the hands up to the shoulders.

- Apply enough pressure to release tension but ensure that the strokes remain flowing and smooth.

- For the forearms, use circular motions with your thumbs and gentle kneading.

- Work your way down the arms and hands, applying more oil as necessary.

Step 4: Focus on the Chest and Abdomen

1. Chest Massage:

- With a generous amount of oil, use circular strokes to massage the chest area, moving outward from the center of the chest toward the armpits.

- Gently massage the sternum, collarbone, and ribs to enhance circulation and promote relaxation.

2. Abdomen Massage:

- Begin by massaging the abdomen in a clockwise direction, following the natural path of digestion.

- Use gentle, clockwise circular strokes, working from the right side of the abdomen, around to the left, and then down to the lower abdomen.

- This promotes digestion and helps relieve tension in the stomach area.

Step 5: Massage the Legs

1. Thighs:

- Using long, sweeping strokes, start at the feet and work your way up the thighs towards the hips.

- Apply gentle kneading motions around the thighs to release any stiffness.

- Focus on areas of tension, such as the hamstrings, by using circular or back-and-forth motions with your palms and fingers.

2. Knees and Calves:

- Massage the knees with circular movements, avoiding direct pressure on the knee joint.

- Continue down the lower legs, using long strokes to stimulate circulation.

- Massage the calves gently with kneading strokes, paying attention to areas of tension.

3. Feet:

- Massage each foot individually, using gentle but firm pressure along the soles and toes.

- Use your thumbs to apply pressure to the arch of the foot, as this can release tension throughout the body.

- Finish by gently stretching the toes and ankles to promote relaxation.

Step 6: Finish with the Back

1. Back Strokes:

- Start at the lower back and work your way up to the shoulders with long, fluid strokes.

- Use both hands in a smooth, rhythmic motion to apply oil to the back, ensuring even coverage.

- Apply more oil as needed to maintain smooth, flowing strokes.

2. Kneading the Lower Back:

- Use your palms and fingers to knead the muscles along the lower back, focusing on tight areas or knots.

- Use circular motions to work out any tension and encourage relaxation.

3. Final Strokes:

- Finish the session with light effleurage (long, sweeping strokes) over the back, shoulders, and limbs to ensure the massage is calming and soothing.

Tips and Variations

- Use gentle pressure, increasing as needed for areas like the shoulders and lower back.

- Focus on areas of tension or discomfort.

- Use circular motions for joints and long strokes for limbs.

- Massage in the direction of hair growth on your scalp and face.

- Avoid massaging over wounds, broken skin, or sensitive areas.

- For Vata constitution, use warming oils like sesame or coconut. For Pitta constitution, use cooling oils like coconut or aloe vera. For Kapha constitution, use drying oils like sesame or sunflower.

- For dry skin, use a moisturizing oil like coconut or olive. For oily skin, use a drying oil like sesame or sunflower.

Aftercare

- Let the oil absorb: Allow the oil to absorb into your skin for 15-30 minutes before showering or bathing.

- Shower or bathe: Use warm water to rinse off excess oil, avoiding hot water, which can strip the skin of its natural oils.

- Moisturize: Apply a gentle moisturizer to lock in the benefits of the Abhyanga oil massage.

Benefits of Abhyanga Oil Massage

Abhyanga offers numerous physical, mental, and emotional benefits, making it a holistic practice that nourishes the body and soul.

1. Promotes Relaxation and Reduces Stress

The rhythmic strokes and warm oils in Abhyanga help soothe the nervous system, reduce stress, and promote a deep sense of relaxation. The massage stimulates the release of endorphins, which are the body's natural stress relievers.

2. Nourishes the Skin

The oils used in Abhyanga are rich in nutrients and antioxidants that hydrate and nourish the skin, leaving it soft, smooth, and glowing. Regular Abhyanga massages can improve the appearance and elasticity of the skin.

3. Enhances Circulation and Detoxification

The massaging technique increases blood flow and promotes the movement of lymphatic fluid, which helps flush out toxins from the body. This enhanced circulation can lead to improved vitality and energy.

4. Balances the Doshas

Abhyanga helps restore balance to the body's three doshas, addressing physical and emotional imbalances that can cause health issues like anxiety, digestive problems, or fatigue.

5. Promotes Better Sleep

The calming nature of the massage helps promote better sleep by reducing tension in the body and calming the mind.

6. Strengthens the Immune System

By promoting detoxification and enhancing circulation, Abhyanga helps strengthen the immune system, making it easier for the body to fight off illnesses.

The Types of Oils Used in Abhyanga

In Abhyanga, the choice of oil plays a crucial role in the overall effectiveness of the massage. Different oils are chosen based on the person's dosha, current health concerns, and the season.

1. Sesame Oil

- **Best for:** Vata dosha (dry, cold, and light constitution).

- **Properties:** Warming, grounding, and nourishing. Sesame oil is commonly used in Abhyanga due to its deep-penetrating and moisturizing properties.

2. Coconut Oil

- **Best for:** Pitta dosha (hot, fiery, and intense constitution).

- **Properties:** Cooling and soothing. Coconut oil is ideal for individuals with sensitive or inflamed skin, offering hydration without excess heat.

3. Mustard Oil

- **Best for:** Kapha dosha (heavy, slow, and cool constitution).

- **Properties:** Warming and stimulating. Mustard oil helps invigorate and energize the body, making it ideal for people feeling sluggish or needing to clear congestion.

4. Almond Oil

- **Best for:** All doshas, especially dry skin.

- **Properties:** Light, nourishing, and calming. Almond oil is great for skin rejuvenation and helps to soothe irritation while moisturizing the skin.

5. Ayurvedic Herbal Oils

- **Best for:** Specific health concerns or imbalances.

- **Properties:** Custom-blended oils contain herbs like turmeric, neem, and brahmi, which are chosen for their therapeutic properties. These oils are used to address specific conditions like inflammation, joint pain, or skin issues.

When to Avoid Abhyanga Oil Massage

While Abhyanga is a safe and beneficial practice for most people, there are a few situations where it may not be suitable:

- If you have certain skin conditions like eczema, rashes, or open wounds.

- If you are experiencing an active infection or inflammation.

- During acute illness or fever, as Abhyanga can increase circulation and potentially exacerbate symptoms.

Conclusion

Abhyanga oil massage is an ancient and deeply restorative practice that nurtures both body and mind. By using warm, medicinal oils and applying gentle strokes to the body, it encourages detoxification, balances the doshas, and promotes overall wellness. Whether performed at home or by a trained practitioner, Abhyanga is a beautiful way to care for your body, reduce stress, and enhance your health, inside and out.

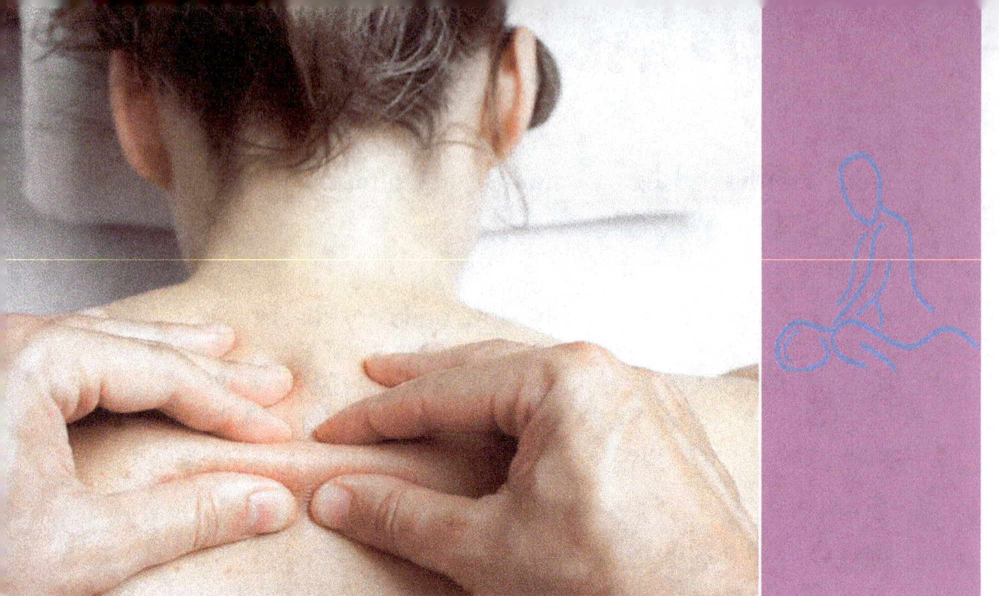

19

MYOFASCIAL RELEASE THERAPY

◇ WHAT IS MYOFASCIAL RELEASE THERAPY?

◇ HOW MYOFASCIAL RELEASE THERAPY WORKS

◇ TECHNIQUES OF MYOFASCIAL RELEASE THERAPY

◇ STEP-BY-STEP MYOFASCIAL RELEASE THERAPY

◇ BENEFITS OF MYOFASCIAL RELEASE THERAPY

Myofascial Release (MFR) is a hands-on technique that focuses on relieving tension in the fascial system, which encompasses the connective tissue surrounding muscles, bones, and organs. This therapy is particularly effective in addressing chronic pain, muscle tightness, and restricted movement, by targeting the fascia—the web-like tissue that connects and supports everything in your body.

In this chapter, we will explore what Myofascial Release Therapy is, how it works, its benefits, techniques, and how it can be integrated into a holistic healing practice.

What is Myofascial Release Therapy?

The fascia is a connective tissue that surrounds and supports muscles, organs, and other structures throughout the body. Over time, this tissue can become tight or restricted due to injury, poor posture, repetitive motion, stress, or trauma. When fascia becomes tight or "locked," it can lead to discomfort, muscle pain, stiffness, and restricted movement.

Myofascial Release Therapy is a form of manual therapy that targets these restrictions in the fascia, using slow, sustained pressure to release the tension and restore mobility. The technique is often used to treat chronic pain, improve flexibility, and promote healing in areas affected by muscular imbalances.

The Fascia and Its Role in the Body

Fascia is more than just a passive tissue—it's a dynamic and essential component of the body. It's made of collagen and elastin fibers, which give it both strength and flexibility. Fascia serves several key roles in the body:

- **Support:** Fascia provides structural support, holding muscles and organs in place.

- **Movement:** It allows muscles to slide smoothly over one another during movement.

- **Protection:** Fascia acts as a protective barrier, cushioning the muscles, bones, and organs it surrounds.

- **Communication:** Fascia is interconnected throughout the body, and tightness in one area can affect distant parts of the body.

The Causes of Myofascial Pain and Restrictions

There are several factors that can lead to myofascial pain and restriction:

- **Trauma or Injury:** A fall, car accident, or sports injury can result in localized trauma that causes the fascia to tighten around the affected area.

- **Repetitive Movements:** Performing the same motions repeatedly—such as sitting at a desk all day or lifting heavy objects—can lead to chronic muscle strain and tension in the fascia.

- **Postural Imbalances:** Poor posture can result in uneven distribution of weight, leading to tension in specific muscle groups and corresponding fascia.

- **Stress:** Mental and emotional stress can cause the muscles to tighten and pull on the fascia, creating pain and discomfort.

- **Scar Tissue:** After an injury, scar tissue can form in the fascia, creating areas of restriction that can affect range of motion.

How Myofascial Release Therapy Works

Myofascial Release Therapy targets the fascia using sustained pressure and gentle stretching. The goal is to release tightness, improve blood flow, and restore the proper movement of muscles and other tissues.

1. Sustained Pressure:

The therapist uses their hands or fingers to apply gentle, sustained pressure to restricted areas of fascia. The pressure is typically held for 90 seconds to 2 minutes at a time, allowing the fascia to relax and lengthen.

2. Gentle Stretching:

After applying pressure, the therapist may use slow, controlled stretching to release the fascial restrictions and improve flexibility.

3. Release of Tension:

As the fascia releases tension, it allows the underlying muscles to relax, which can reduce pain and improve movement.

Techniques of Myofascial Release Therapy

Myofascial Release Therapy utilizes several specific techniques to target fascial restrictions. These techniques are typically customized to address the specific needs of each client. Here are some of the most commonly used methods:

1. Direct Myofascial Release:

This technique involves applying direct, sustained pressure to areas of fascial restriction. The therapist uses their hands or fingers to "sink" into the tissue and hold the pressure until the fascia begins to release and lengthen.

2. Indirect Myofascial Release:

In this technique, the therapist uses a more gentle touch to move the fascia in the direction it wants to go. It is particularly useful when working with sensitive or injured tissue.

3. Myofascial Stretching:

Myofascial stretching involves gently elongating the fascia to promote better flexibility. It is often combined with other techniques to release tension and improve range of motion.

4. Trigger Point Therapy:

Trigger points are tight knots in muscles that can cause pain in other areas of the body. MFR therapists may incorporate trigger point therapy to release muscle knots and alleviate referred pain.

Step-by-Step Myofascial Release Therapy Guide

Here is a step-by-step guide for performing myofascial release therapy:

Preparation

1. **Consultation:**

   - Before starting the therapy, ask the client about their pain history, specific areas of discomfort, and any conditions that may contraindicate myofascial release, such as recent injuries or inflammation.

   - Discuss any areas of chronic tension, stiffness, or muscle imbalances that the client would like to address.

2. Create a Comfortable Environment:

- Ensure the room is quiet, warm, and free from distractions to promote relaxation.

- Consider using soft, calming music and dim lighting.

3. Prepare the Client:

- Have the client lie comfortably on a massage table or in a position that allows easy access to the areas of tension (such as on their back, stomach, or side, depending on the targeted area).

- Ensure the client is properly draped and comfortable.

4. Warm Up the Tissue (Optional):

- Before starting myofascial release, you may perform a few minutes of general effleurage (light, smooth strokes) to warm up the muscles and fascia. This helps prepare the body for deeper work.

Step 1: Identify Areas of Tension

1. Assess the Body:

- Begin by gently palpating the areas of tension or discomfort. Use your fingers, palms, or forearms to feel for tight, rope-like bands in the fascia or muscles.

- Pay close attention to the client's feedback regarding sensitivity or areas of greater discomfort.

2. Find Myofascial Restrictions:

- Myofascial restrictions often feel like tight bands, nodules, or "knots" in the muscle tissue. These areas of tension can cause pain and limit movement.

- Once a restricted area is located, focus on it for the next steps in the therapy.

Step 2: Apply Gentle, Sustained Pressure

1. Gentle Stretching of the Fascia:

- Use slow, deliberate pressure to apply gentle stretch to the fascia. Unlike traditional massage, myofascial release doesn't involve fast or repetitive strokes.

•	Apply steady, sustained pressure to the area for 90 seconds to 2 minutes, allowing the tissue to gradually soften and release.

2. Use the Palm or Thumb:

•	For larger areas (like the back or thighs), use the palm or flat of your hand. For more focused areas (like the shoulders or neck), use your thumb, fingers, or elbow for deeper pressure.

•	Maintain a constant amount of pressure, and allow the tissue to slowly yield to your touch. Do not rush this step.

3. Monitor the Client's Response:

•	Check in with the client throughout the process to ensure the pressure is comfortable and they are not experiencing pain. The pressure should be strong enough to create a sense of deep stretch but should not be painful.

Step 3: Engage in the Release of Tension

1. Allow the Fascia to "Release":

•	While holding pressure on a restricted area, the fascia will often begin to "release" after some time. You may feel the tissue soften, loosen, or even shift under your hands.

•	You may notice the client's muscles relax, or they may experience a sense of lightness or relief as the fascia begins to lengthen and become more pliable.

2. Gentle Stretching Movements:

•	After holding pressure on a restricted area, gently move the tissue to further enhance the release. For example, you might stretch the muscle in the opposite direction of the restriction or use small oscillating motions to help ease the fascia.

3. Encourage Breathing:

•	Remind the client to breathe deeply and slowly throughout the session. Breathing deeply helps to relax the body and facilitates the release of tension.

•	Encourage exhalation during moments of deeper pressure, as this helps the body relax further.

Step 4: Move to Adjacent Areas

1. Work on Adjacent Muscles and Fascia:

- After releasing tension in one area, move to nearby muscles and fascia. The fascia is interconnected, so releasing tension in one area often leads to improvements in adjacent areas.

- For example, if you're working on the lower back, you may move to the glutes, hamstrings, or even the feet, as these areas are often affected by myofascial restrictions in the back.

2. Use Long Strokes or Cross-Fiber Friction:

- For larger areas, use long, flowing strokes along the muscle fibers to enhance circulation and help release general tightness.

- For more localized restrictions, you can use cross-fiber friction, which involves applying pressure perpendicular to the muscle fibers to help break up scar tissue or adhesions.

Step 5: Stretch and Reassess

1. Passive Stretching:

- After working on an area, you can gently stretch the client's muscles to help further release tension. For example, you can stretch the arms, legs, or neck in the direction opposite of the tension you just released.

- Hold the stretch for 15–30 seconds, allowing the muscles and fascia to lengthen and release.

2. Reassess the Area:

- After working on one area, check in with the client to see if the tension has been reduced. Use your hands to palpate the area again and notice any changes in the texture, temperature, or tightness of the tissue.

3. Repeat as Necessary:

- Myofascial release may need to be repeated on different areas of the body, especially in cases of chronic tightness or pain. Take your time and work slowly and systematically through the body.

Step 6: Finish the Session with Gentle Techniques

1. Gentle Effleurage:

- At the end of the session, use gentle effleurage (long, smooth strokes) to calm the body and promote circulation. This helps to disperse any remaining tension and leaves the client feeling relaxed.

- Apply lighter strokes toward the heart to support lymphatic circulation.

2. Final Stretching:

- Use gentle stretching movements for the muscles that were worked during the session. These stretches should be slow and controlled to ensure they are effective but not too intense.

Step 7: Aftercare and Recommendations

1. Hydrate:

- Encourage the client to drink plenty of water after the session to help flush out toxins and prevent any soreness.

- Myofascial release can cause the release of metabolic waste products, so hydration is important.

2. Rest:

- Advise the client to rest after the session to allow the body time to absorb the benefits. If they feel any soreness, this is often a sign that the therapy is working to release deep-held tension.

3. Follow-up Sessions:

- For chronic tension or pain, it may take several sessions to fully release restrictions in the fascia. Suggest a regular schedule based on the client's needs and response to the therapy.

Important Considerations

- **Gentle Pressure:** Myofascial release involves applying sustained pressure to the fascia, but the pressure should never cause pain. If the client experiences sharp or intense pain, reduce the pressure immediately.

- **Slow and Steady:** This technique is not about quick, intense movements but rather about slow, deliberate pressure to release deep-held tension. Give each area enough time to respond to the release.

- **Communication:** Regularly check in with the client to ensure they are comfortable, especially if you are applying deep pressure.

Benefits of Myofascial Release Therapy

1. Pain Relief:

One of the most common reasons people seek Myofascial Release is to relieve chronic pain. By targeting fascial restrictions, the therapy reduces muscle tightness, eases discomfort, and helps alleviate pain from conditions like fibromyalgia, chronic back pain, and sciatica.

2. Improved Range of Motion:

Myofascial Release helps restore flexibility by releasing tension in the fascia and muscles. This is especially beneficial for people with limited movement due to injuries or chronic conditions.

3. Better Posture:

By releasing tension in areas affected by poor posture (such as the neck, back, and shoulders), MFR can improve alignment and reduce the risk of future postural problems.

4. Increased Blood Flow and Circulation:

The sustained pressure applied during the therapy promotes better circulation, helping to remove waste products from the muscles and deliver oxygen and nutrients.

5. Stress Reduction:

Myofascial Release is deeply relaxing, helping to release physical tension and, by extension, mental and emotional stress.

6. Enhanced Healing:

Myofascial Release can promote the healing of scar tissue, improve muscle recovery after injury, and support overall tissue repair.

Who Can Benefit from Myofascial Release Therapy?

1. People with Chronic Pain:

Those suffering from conditions like fibromyalgia, arthritis, or chronic back pain can benefit greatly from Myofascial Release.

2. Athletes and Active Individuals:
Athletes or those who engage in regular physical activity often experience muscle tightness and fascial restrictions. MFR can help with recovery, flexibility, and performance.

3. Individuals with Postural Problems:
If you spend long hours sitting at a desk or have poor posture, MFR can help relieve the tension in your back, neck, and shoulders.

4. People Recovering from Injury or Surgery:
MFR is effective for healing after an injury or surgery, as it helps reduce scar tissue and promotes muscle recovery.

5. Those Seeking Stress Relief:
Since Myofascial Release helps reduce stress and promote relaxation, it is also beneficial for those seeking relief from the physical effects of mental stress.

Contraindications for Myofascial Release Therapy

While Myofascial Release is generally safe for most individuals, there are certain situations where it may not be recommended:

- **Acute injuries** with inflammation or swelling.

- **Osteoporosis** or bone conditions where deep pressure could cause harm.

- **Infections** or areas of active infection.

- **Cancer** in the area being treated.

Conclusion

Myofascial Release Therapy is an incredibly effective technique for addressing the root cause of chronic pain, stiffness, and limited movement. By targeting restrictions in the fascia, this therapy helps promote relaxation, improve flexibility, and accelerate the body's healing process. Whether used to address specific injuries, reduce tension, or improve overall mobility, Myofascial Release is a powerful tool in restoring balance and comfort to the body.

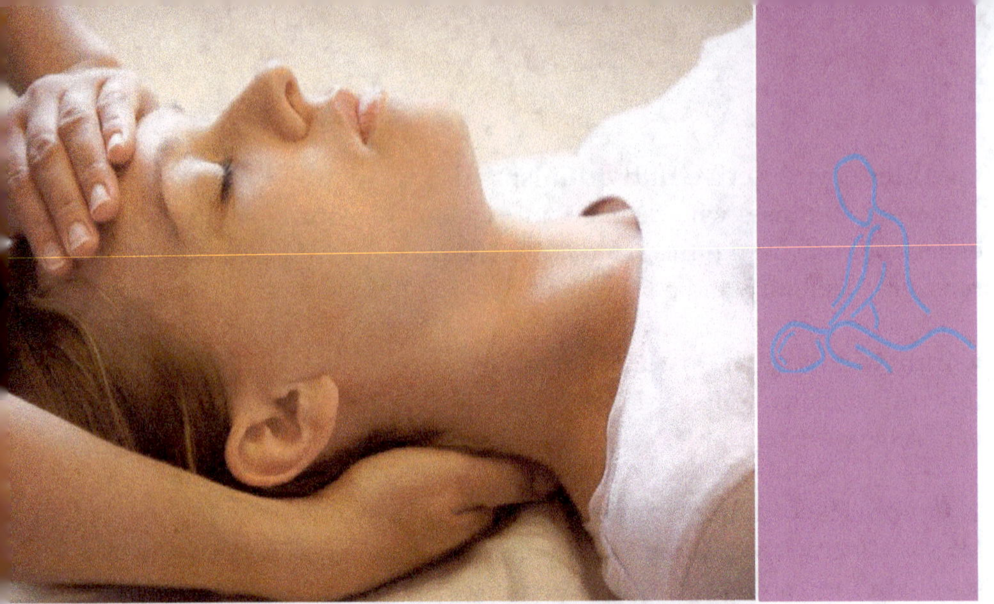

20

CRANIOSACRAL THERAPY

 **WHAT YOU'LL LEARN** 

◊ WHAT IS CRANIOSACRAL THERAPY?

◊ HOW DOES CRANIOSACRAL THERAPY WORK?

◊ TECHNIQUES IN CRANIOSACRAL THERAPY

◊ STEP-BY-STEP CRANIOSACRAL THERAPY

◊ BENEFITS OF CRANIOSACRAL THERAPY

◊ CONDITIONS TREATED WITH CRANIOSACRAL

THERAPY

Craniosacral Therapy (CST) is a gentle, non-invasive treatment method that focuses on the cerebrospinal fluid and the structures that surround the brain and spinal cord. Using light touch and subtle techniques, CST aims to relieve restrictions, balance the craniosacral rhythm, and promote overall healing throughout the body.

This therapy is rooted in the idea that the flow of cerebrospinal fluid—the fluid that surrounds the brain and spinal cord—affects the body's physical and emotional health. Through CST, practitioners can address underlying tensions and imbalances, helping to improve physical function, relieve stress, and enhance emotional well-being.

What is Craniosacral Therapy?

Craniosacral Therapy is a hands-on healing technique that targets the soft tissues and fluid surrounding the brain and spinal cord, collectively known as the craniosacral system. This system plays a crucial role in the central nervous system, helping to protect, nourish, and support the brain and spinal cord.

The therapy is based on the idea that the body's craniosacral rhythm (a subtle, rhythmic movement of the cerebrospinal fluid) can become disrupted due to injury, trauma, stress, or disease. By gently applying light touch to various points along the body, especially the head, neck, and spine, CST practitioners help to release restrictions and restore balance to the craniosacral system, leading to overall health improvements.

The History and Foundations of Craniosacral Therapy

Craniosacral Therapy was developed by Dr. John Upledger, an osteopathic physician, in the 1970s. Dr. Upledger's research revealed that the craniosacral system could be palpated, and he began to understand how its rhythm could be assessed and manipulated for therapeutic purposes. He combined osteopathic principles with techniques aimed at balancing the body's fluids and energy systems, which led to the development of CST.

The foundational concept behind CST is that the body has its own innate ability to heal, and by working with the craniosacral rhythm, practitioners can facilitate this healing process. It is a holistic therapy that connects the body, mind, and spirit, addressing physical, emotional, and energetic imbalances.

How Does Craniosacral Therapy Work?

The primary technique used in Craniosacral Therapy is a very light touch (usually no more than 5 grams of pressure, roughly the weight of a nickel). Practitioners assess the craniosacral rhythm and apply gentle pressure to specific areas of the body, including the head, neck, spine, and sacrum (the base of the spine).

1. The Craniosacral Rhythm

The cerebrospinal fluid, which is produced in the brain's ventricles, circulates around the brain and spinal cord. As it moves through the central nervous system, it creates a subtle rhythm. This rhythm is key to the body's healing process and is closely connected to the function of the entire nervous system. CST practitioners can feel this rhythmic movement and use it to guide their therapeutic touch.

2. Releasing Tension

When the craniosacral rhythm becomes impaired or restricted (due to trauma, injury, emotional stress, or illness), the body can develop tension patterns that may manifest as pain, discomfort, or other dysfunctions. CST works by gently releasing these restrictions, allowing the cerebrospinal fluid to flow freely and restore balance.

3. Supporting the Nervous System

CST helps improve the overall functioning of the nervous system by ensuring that the brain and spinal cord are adequately nourished, protected, and supported. By alleviating blockages and improving circulation, CST promotes better communication between the brain and the rest of the body.

Techniques in Craniosacral Therapy

CST techniques are highly specialized, and each session is tailored to the individual's needs. Below are some key techniques commonly used during Craniosacral Therapy:

1. Cranial Manipulation

This technique focuses on gently adjusting the bones of the skull, which are thought to have slight mobility. These gentle manipulations can help release tension and restore balance to the craniosacral system.

2. Sacral Touch

A key focus of CST is the sacrum (the bone at the base of the spine). By applying gentle pressure to the sacrum, the practitioner can release tension throughout the entire spine and pelvis.

3. Fascia Release

The fascia is a connective tissue that surrounds muscles, organs, and nerves. CST practitioners may use gentle pressure to release restrictions in the fascia, which can improve circulation and mobility.

4. Diaphragm Release

Since the diaphragm plays a central role in respiration, CST can include techniques aimed at releasing tension in the diaphragm. This can help improve breath flow, ease tension in the upper body, and support better respiratory health.

Step-by-Step Guide to Craniosacral Therapy

Here is a step-by-step guide to performing a Craniosacral Therapy session.

Preparation

1. **Set Up a Calm Environment**

   - Choose a quiet, comfortable space with minimal distractions.

   - Dim the lighting and consider using soothing music or aromatherapy to enhance relaxation.

2. **Prepare Yourself**

   - Ground yourself through a few deep breaths or a brief meditation to center your focus.

   - Ensure your hands are warm and free of any lotions or oils, as they are not typically used in CST.

3. **Position the Client**

   - Have the client lie on their back on a massage table, fully clothed.

   - Provide pillows or bolsters to support their neck, knees, or lower back for comfort.

Step 1: Establish Connection

- **Light Touch Assessment:** Place your hands gently on the client's head, shoulders, or feet to tune into their craniosacral rhythm.

- **Feel for Subtle Rhythms:** Pay attention to the movement of the cerebrospinal fluid. It may feel like a gentle pulse or wave beneath your hands.

- Take your time to become attuned to the client's body and establish trust.

Step 2: Address the Head (Cranial Area)

1. Base of the Skull (Occipital Hold):

- Gently cup the base of the skull with both hands.

- Allow your hands to feel the natural movement of the occiput and wait for signs of relaxation or release.

2. Forehead and Crown (Frontal Hold):

- Place one hand on the forehead and the other on the back of the head.

- Feel for any restrictions or imbalances in the cranial movement and gently support the body's natural adjustments.

3. Temporal Bones:

- Lightly hold the sides of the head near the ears.

- Sense the motion of the temporal bones and provide subtle encouragement for balance.

Step 3: Address the Spine and Sacrum

1. Neck and Upper Spine:

- Move your hands to the base of the neck.

- Feel for restrictions and allow the body to unwind naturally.

2. Lower Spine and Sacrum:

- Place one hand under the sacrum (the triangular bone at the base of the spine).

- Support the sacrum's subtle movement and allow the body to release tension in this area.

Step 4: Full-Body Integration

- Place one hand on the client's head and the other on their feet.

- Sense the entire craniosacral rhythm, helping the body to synchronize and harmonize.

- Hold this position for several minutes, allowing the client's body to enter a deep state of relaxation and integration.

Step 5: Conclude the Session

1. **Transition Gently:**

- Slowly lift your hands from the client's body to end the physical connection.

- Allow the client to remain still for a few moments before sitting up.

2. **Post-Session Feedback:**

- Share any observations with the client and invite them to express how they feel.

- Offer advice for continued relaxation, such as staying hydrated and avoiding strenuous activity immediately after the session.

Tips for Effective Craniosacral Therapy

- **Patience is Key:** CST is a subtle therapy. Allow time for the client's body to respond to your touch.

- **Stay Neutral:** Avoid imposing force or intention; simply follow the body's natural rhythms and cues.

- **Practice Mindfulness:** Maintain a calm, focused presence throughout the session to create a safe and healing space for the client.

By following these steps, Craniosacral Therapy can become a profound tool for relaxation, healing, and balance, benefiting both the practitioner and the client.

Benefits of Craniosacral Therapy

Craniosacral Therapy has a wide range of benefits for both physical and emotional health. These benefits can vary depending on individual needs, but some of the most commonly reported outcomes include:

1. Pain Relief

CST is often used to alleviate chronic pain, especially in the neck, back, and head. It can help relieve headaches, migraines, and tension, as well as reduce discomfort related to conditions such as fibromyalgia and temporomandibular joint (TMJ) disorder.

2. Stress Reduction and Emotional Healing

Because of its gentle and soothing nature, CST is highly effective in reducing stress, anxiety, and emotional tension. By calming the nervous system, CST can help release trapped emotions and promote a deep sense of relaxation. Many clients report feeling more grounded, centered, and emotionally balanced after a session.

3. Improved Mobility and Flexibility

By releasing restrictions in the craniosacral system, CST can help improve mobility and flexibility, especially in the neck, shoulders, and spine. This can lead to a better range of motion and improved posture.

4. Enhanced Brain and Spinal Health

Since CST works directly with the brain and spinal cord, it can support overall nervous system function, enhance mental clarity, and improve cognitive function. CST is also used to help with conditions such as brain fog, learning difficulties, and concentration issues.

5. Boosted Immune System

Craniosacral Therapy encourages better circulation of cerebrospinal fluid, which nourishes the brain and spinal cord. This improves overall health and helps strengthen the immune system, allowing the body to fight off illness and maintain optimal function.

6. Relief for Traumatic Injuries

CST can be particularly beneficial for individuals recovering from traumatic injuries (such as car accidents or falls), surgery, or childbirth. The therapy promotes healing and reduces the lasting effects of trauma by addressing both the physical and emotional aspects of the injury.

Conditions Treated with Craniosacral Therapy

Craniosacral Therapy can be used to address a wide range of conditions, both physical and emotional. Common conditions treated with CST include:

- Headaches and Migraines

- Neck and Back Pain

- Stress and Anxiety

- Chronic Fatigue

- TMJ (Temporomandibular Joint) Dysfunction

- Fibromyalgia

- Post-Traumatic Stress Disorder (PTSD)

- Concussions and Brain Injuries

- Insomnia and Sleep Disorders

- Digestive Disorders

- Reproductive Health Issues

- Pediatric Conditions (e.g., colic, ear infections)

How to Experience Craniosacral Therapy

Craniosacral Therapy is typically performed in a comfortable, quiet setting. The client lies fully clothed on a massage table while the practitioner uses gentle touch to assess and manipulate the craniosacral system. Sessions typically last between 30 minutes to an hour, and many people experience a deep sense of relaxation and calm during and after treatment.

Conclusion

Craniosacral Therapy is a powerful yet gentle therapeutic technique that promotes healing and restores balance in the body's central nervous system. By working with the craniosacral rhythm and addressing restrictions in the brain, spine, and surrounding tissues, CST can provide relief from chronic pain, stress, emotional tension, and many other health concerns. Whether you're seeking relief from a specific condition or simply looking for relaxation and overall wellness, Craniosacral Therapy offers a holistic, nurturing approach to health and healing.

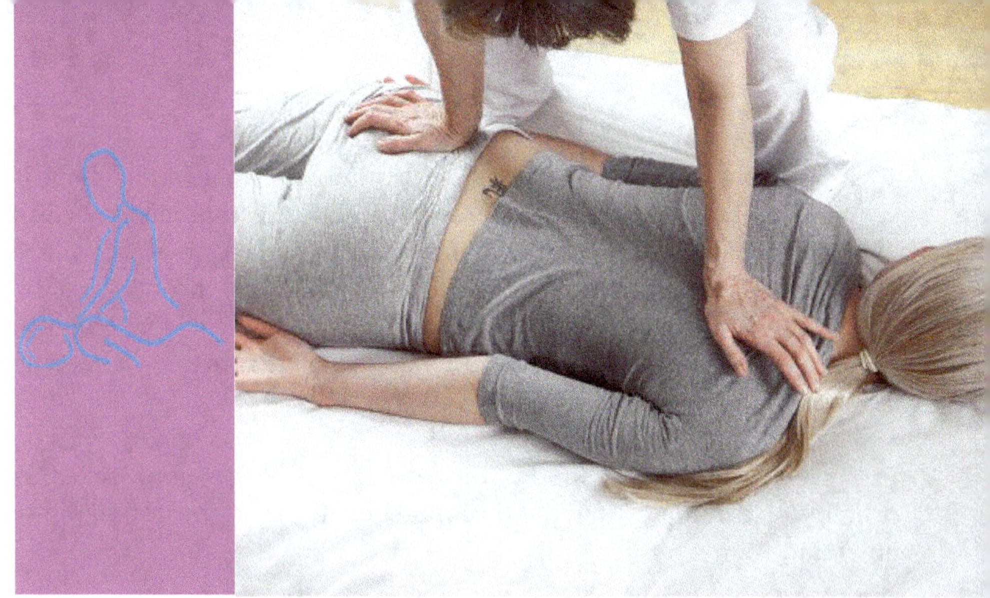

21

SHIATSU MASSAGE

WHAT YOU'LL LEARN

◊ UNDERSTANDING THE PRINCIPLES OF SHIATSU

◊ TECHNIQUES OF SHIATSU MASSAGE

◊ STEP-BY-STEP SHIATSU MASSAGE

◊ BENEFITS OF SHIATSU MASSAGE

Shiatsu massage, a cornerstone of traditional Japanese healing, is much more than a physical therapy; it's a holistic approach to health and well-being. Rooted in the principles of Traditional Chinese Medicine (TCM), Shiatsu focuses on stimulating energy flow (qi) through specific pathways called meridians. This ancient practice helps restore balance, relieve tension, and promote relaxation, making it a versatile and deeply restorative massage technique.

In this chapter, we'll explore the essence of Shiatsu massage, its principles, techniques, and the profound benefits it offers for both body and mind.

Understanding the Principles of Shiatsu

Shiatsu, which translates to "finger pressure," is a therapy that emphasizes the connection between physical touch and energetic flow. Practitioners believe that disruptions in the flow of qi can lead to physical discomfort, emotional imbalances, and illness. By applying targeted pressure along the body's meridians, Shiatsu works to unblock these energy pathways, supporting the body's natural ability to heal itself.

Key Concepts in Shiatsu

1. Meridians and Energy Flow:

The body has twelve primary meridians, each associated with specific organs and functions. Shiatsu aims to harmonize these energy channels, promoting overall vitality.

2. Pressure and Touch:

Unlike other massage styles, Shiatsu uses finger, thumb, palm, and sometimes elbow pressure to stimulate energy points. The intensity of pressure is adjusted based on the recipient's needs, creating a tailored and effective experience.

3.Holistic Approach:

Shiatsu doesn't just address physical symptoms; it considers the emotional and spiritual aspects of health. By restoring energy flow, it supports mental clarity and emotional balance.

Techniques of Shiatsu Massage

Shiatsu incorporates a variety of techniques to address tension, discomfort, and energy blockages. These techniques are applied with care, ensuring the client feels both relaxed and rejuvenated.

1. Applying Pressure to Acupressure Points

Pressure is the foundation of Shiatsu. Practitioners use their fingers, thumbs, or palms to press on specific points along the meridians. These points, known as acupressure points, correspond to various organs and systems in the body.

- **Gentle Yet Firm Touch:** Pressure is applied steadily and released slowly, creating a soothing and grounding effect.

- **Tailored Intensity:** The practitioner adjusts the intensity based on the client's preferences and the areas being treated.

2. Stretching and Mobilization

Stretching helps to release tension and improve flexibility. Common stretches include:

- Gently pulling and stretching the arms and legs.

- Rotating joints such as shoulders, wrists, and ankles.

- Spinal twists to relieve back tension and enhance mobility.

3. Rhythmic Movements

Shiatsu often involves rhythmic, wave-like movements that mirror the natural flow of energy. These movements:

- Encourage relaxation.

- Stimulate circulation.

- Support the release of physical and emotional stress.

4. Breathing and Energy Synchronization

Both the client and the practitioner focus on deep, rhythmic breathing. Synchronizing the pressure and movements with the client's breath enhances the therapy's effectiveness and helps deepen relaxation.

Step-by-Step Guide to Shiatsu Massage

Below is a step-by-step guide to performing a Shiatsu massage.

Preparation

1. Create a Suitable Environment

• Select a quiet, clean, and calm space with enough room for the client to lie on a futon or mat on the floor (the traditional setup).

• Ensure a relaxing atmosphere with soft lighting and optional soothing music.

2. Prepare Yourself

• Center yourself through deep breathing or a brief meditation to focus your energy.

• Warm up your hands and ensure you're in comfortable, loose-fitting clothing, as Shiatsu involves movement.

3. Position the Client

• The client remains fully clothed and lies down on their back.

• Encourage them to relax and breathe deeply.

Step 1: Grounding and Initial Assessment

• **Establish Connection:** Place your hands gently on the client's shoulders or abdomen to connect and feel their energy.

• **Observe the Body:** Pay attention to areas of tension or imbalance as you lightly press along the client's body.

Step 2: Work on the Meridian Lines

Shiatsu focuses on stimulating energy pathways (meridians). Apply gentle, consistent pressure using your fingers, thumbs, palms, or elbows along the following meridian areas:

1. Head and Neck:

• Use your thumbs to press gently on points along the scalp, temples, and base of the skull.

• Massage around the neck, focusing on releasing tension and promoting relaxation.

2. Shoulders and Arms:

• Apply thumb pressure to the tops of the shoulders and along the outer arms.

• Stretch the arms gently to relieve stiffness.

3. Back (if the client is lying face down):

- Use your palms or knuckles to press along both sides of the spine.

- Work on the upper back and shoulder blades to release knots and tension.

4. Chest and Abdomen:

- Use light, circular pressure on points around the chest and abdomen.

- Encourage the client to breathe deeply to aid relaxation.

5. Legs and Feet:

- Apply thumb pressure along the outer and inner thighs, calves, and shins.

- Focus on acupressure points around the ankles and soles of the feet to stimulate energy flow.

Step 3: Stretching and Mobilization

1. Passive Stretching:

- Gently move the client's limbs to stretch the muscles and joints.

- For example, lift and stretch the legs while applying light pressure to the thighs.

2. Rotations:

- Rotate the shoulders, wrists, ankles, and hips in a controlled and smooth motion to increase flexibility and mobility.

3. Spinal Stretches:

- If appropriate, guide the client into a gentle spinal twist or stretch to release tension along the back.

Step 4: Focus on Key Acupressure Points

Shiatsu incorporates specific points to address common issues like stress, fatigue, and pain:

- **For Stress Relief:** Press gently on the area between the eyebrows and at the base of the skull.

- **For Energy Boost:** Stimulate the point three fingers below the navel (known as the "sea of qi").

- **For Pain Relief:** Apply pressure to the fleshy area between the thumb and index finger.

Step 5: Closure
1. **Harmonize the Body's Energy:**

   - Perform light, sweeping motions across the body to balance the energy flow.

   - Place your hands on the abdomen or shoulders for a final moment of connection.

2. **Conclude the Session:**

   - Encourage the client to rest for a few moments before sitting up.

   - Offer water and remind them to stay hydrated after the session.

Tips for an Effective Shiatsu Massage

- **Pressure Control:** Adjust the pressure according to the client's preference, ensuring it's firm but not painful.

- **Breath Awareness:** Sync your movements with the client's breathing to enhance relaxation.

- **Be Present:** Stay fully focused on the client's needs and responses throughout the session.

By following these steps, Shiatsu massage can become a powerful method to relieve tension, enhance energy flow, and support overall well-being.

Benefits of Shiatsu Massage
Shiatsu massage offers a wide range of benefits for physical, emotional, and mental health.

Physical Benefits

- **Relieves Muscle Tension:** The targeted pressure helps release tight muscles and alleviate pain.

- **Enhances Circulation:** By stimulating the meridians, Shiatsu improves blood flow and supports the body's natural healing processes.

- **Boosts Immunity:** Regular sessions are believed to strengthen the immune system by enhancing the body's energy flow.

Emotional and Mental Benefits

- **Reduces Stress and Anxiety:** The calming touch of Shiatsu creates a sense of grounding and inner peace.

- **Promotes Emotional Balance:** By harmonizing qi, Shiatsu can help release emotional blockages and restore balance.

- **Improves Sleep Quality:** Many clients report better sleep after Shiatsu sessions due to its deeply relaxing effects.

Holistic Well-Being

Shiatsu's emphasis on energy balance means that it doesn't just address immediate symptoms—it supports long-term health by promoting harmony within the body, mind, and spirit.

Is Shiatsu Right for Everyone?

Shiatsu is gentle and non-invasive, making it suitable for most people. However, certain conditions may require caution:

- Pregnancy (consult a professional trained in prenatal massage).

- Recent injuries or surgeries.

- Severe medical conditions (e.g., cancer, heart disease).

Always communicate openly with the practitioner about your health concerns to ensure a safe and beneficial experience.

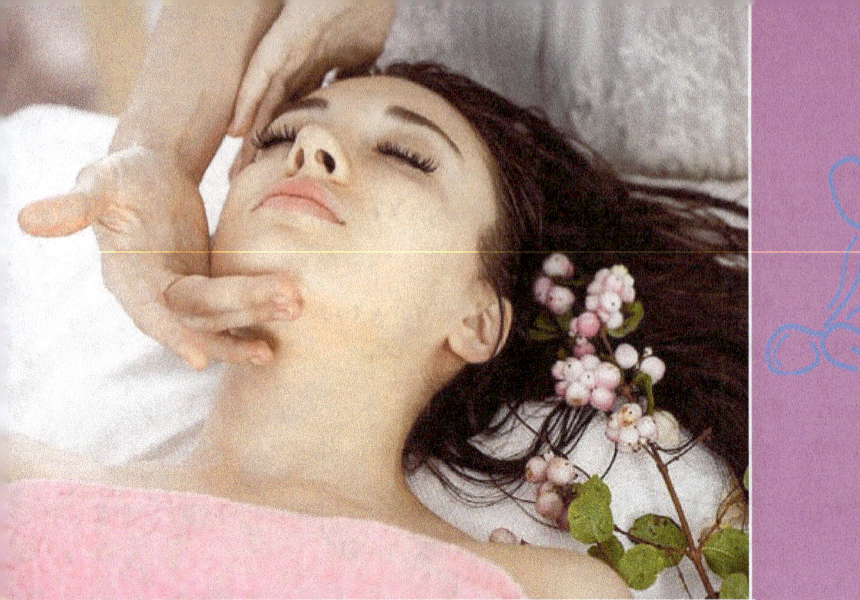

22

ENHANCING SKILLS WITH PRACTICE AND FEEDBACK

WHAT YOU'LL LEARN

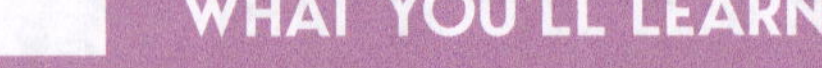

◊ HOW TO PRACTICE ON DIFFERENT PEOPLE

◊ THE ROLE OF FEEDBACK

◊ TIPS FOR DEVELOPING INTUITION AND SENSITIVITY

Refining Your Technique

By now, you've learned the basics of massage techniques, understood the benefits of touch, and begun exploring how massage can help manage stress, pain, and tension. But the journey doesn't end here. Infact, mastering massage is a continuous process of growth, learning, and refinement. This chapter will focus on how to refine your technique, improve your touch, and develop a deeper connection to the body through practice and feedback.

Whether you're a beginner or have been practicing for some time, there's always room for improvement. The path to becoming an exceptional massage therapist is paved with consistent practice, openness to feedback, and a growing sense of intuition. In this chapter, we'll look at how to practice effectively on different people, how to use feedback to enhance your skills, and how to develop sensitivity and intuition in your touch.

How to Practice Effectively on Different People

The first and most essential step in improving your skills is practice. The more you practice, the more you'll understand the nuances of your touch and the various ways people's bodies respond to massage. But practicing doesn't mean you should just go through the motions—it's about actively engaging with different bodies, different needs, and different situations.

Practice on a Variety of People:

One of the best ways to expand your massage expertise is by practicing on different people. Everyone's body is unique, and the more varied your practice, the better you'll be at adapting your touch to suit a wide range of needs. If you practice only on one type of person—say, someone who's very athletic—you might miss out on learning how to adjust for different body types, tension areas, or personal preferences.

Here are some examples of different individuals to practice on:

- **Athletes and Active Individuals:** Working with athletes allows you to address muscle soreness, stiffness, and sports-related injuries. You'll learn to apply more pressure and work through deeper layers of muscle tissue to alleviate post-exercise tension and speed recovery.

- **Older Adults:** Older individuals tend to have more fragile skin and muscles that are less elastic, making gentle pressure and more focused, slow movements essential. Practicing with older clients will help you refine your skills in applying a light touch, particularly for areas such as the lower back, hands, and feet.

- **People with Chronic Pain:** Working with individuals who suffer from chronic conditions like arthritis, fibromyalgia, or muscle pain will teach you how to approach massage with sensitivity. This allows you to experiment with both gentle and more moderate pressure to identify what provides the most relief.

- **Pregnant Clients:** Pregnancy brings unique challenges, and massage can offer immense benefits. Practicing on expectant mothers, under proper guidance, helps you learn how to support their changing body with proper positioning, pressure, and specific techniques.

Pay Attention to Different Body Types:

It's also important to recognize that different body types will respond to touch in different ways. For example, individuals with more muscle mass may require firmer pressure to get into deeper muscle layers, while those with less muscle may prefer a gentler touch. Someone with a lot of tension in their upper back might need more focus in that area, while someone with tension in their lower body may need a different set of techniques.

By practicing on people of varying body types and lifestyles, you'll learn how to adjust your pressure, rhythm, and technique for different needs. This experience will give you the versatility to work with a broad range of clients and their unique preferences.

Adjusting Techniques for Specific Areas:

One of the key things you'll learn from practicing on various people is how to approach different areas of the body. For example, the shoulders and neck often carry a lot of stress, so they may need more time and focus. The lower back and legs might require slower, longer strokes to release built-up tension.

Experimenting with Pressure:

As you practice, pay close attention to how much pressure you're applying. The right amount of pressure can make a world of difference in how effective your massage is. Too little pressure and the client may not feel any relief; too much pressure and they may experience discomfort or even pain. Practicing different pressure techniques—light, moderate, and deep—will help you learn how to adjust according to your client's comfort levels and needs.

The Role of Feedback in Improving Your Touch and Technique

Feedback is a cornerstone of growth as a massage therapist. It allows you to refine your techniques, adjust to your client's preferences, and learn how to better serve their needs. By encouraging honest and constructive feedback, you can continuously improve your practice, and develop a deeper connection with your clients.

The Importance of Active Listening:

One of the most effective ways to gather feedback is simply by listening to your clients. Often, clients may give subtle cues about their comfort levels or the effectiveness of your techniques. For instance, if they tense up when you apply pressure in a specific area, they may be signaling discomfort or asking you to ease up. On the other hand, if they let out a deep sigh or say "that feels great," you know you're on the right track. To maximize the value of feedback, be proactive in asking for it. While some clients will naturally volunteer their thoughts, others may need a little encouragement. After the session, ask them about their experience:

- "How was the pressure? Was it too much or just right?"

- "Did you feel relief in the areas we worked on?"

- "Were there any spots where you felt more tension after the massage?"

- "How do you feel now—more relaxed or still carrying some stress?"

These questions will provide insights into areas where you may need to adjust, such as the pressure, rhythm, or even the duration of your session.

Feedback Doesn't Always Come Immediately:

Sometimes, clients may not immediately know how to express what felt right or wrong during a massage. It's important to let them reflect and follow up after a few hours, especially if they're feeling any soreness or discomfort. They may realize that certain areas feel better or worse as the massage settles into their muscles.

Use Feedback as a Tool for Growth:

Feedback is not only about what you did right but also about where you can improve. For instance, if a client mentions that one technique felt too harsh, or a certain area was not addressed enough, take note of it. Use this feedback to practice and adjust your touch for future sessions. The more you incorporate feedback, the more adept you'll become at providing personalized, effective massages that meet each individual's needs.

Tips for Developing Intuition and Sensitivity as a Massage Therapist

As you continue practicing and receiving feedback, your goal should be to develop a deeper sense of intuition in your touch. Massage therapy goes beyond technique—it involves a subtle connection to the body, and developing a sensitivity to the needs of your clients can take your practice to a whole new level.

Pay Attention to the Sensations Under Your Hands:

One of the most essential ways to develop sensitivity is by paying attention to what your hands are telling you. As you apply pressure to different muscle groups, your hands can feel the resistance, tightness, or release of muscle fibers. This can guide you in knowing when to apply deeper pressure, when to ease off, and when to move on to a different area. Over time, your hands will become attuned to the unique texture and response of each muscle group.

Feel the Rhythm of the Body:

Another aspect of intuition in massage is learning the natural rhythm of the body. The way a muscle contracts and relaxes will tell you how to apply pressure and when to adjust your rhythm. For example, some muscles may respond well to slow, deliberate strokes, while others may need a faster rhythm to increase circulation or promote energy flow. By observing how the body reacts, you'll be able to adjust your technique to create the most effective treatment.

Trusting Your Inner Sense:
As you gain experience, trust your instincts. There will be moments when you intuitively feel that a certain technique is right for the moment or when you sense that a client is holding tension in a specific spot. Trusting this inner sense of touch allows you to tailor each session to meet your client's exact needs. This is where the art of massage truly shines: not only applying learned techniques but also responding organically to the body's signals.

Mindful Awareness:
Mindful awareness is key to developing a deeper connection with your clients. Be present in each session, focusing entirely on the body beneath your hands. This mindfulness allows you to be fully aware of the subtle responses that occur during the massage, such as muscle tightness, temperature changes, and emotional shifts. By practicing mindful touch, you deepen your intuition and refine your sensitivity, making each massage more effective and personalized.

Conclusion

In this chapter, we've discussed how to effectively practice massage on different people, how to incorporate feedback to improve your technique, and how to develop intuition and sensitivity in your touch. Massage is both an art and a science, and through consistent practice, feedback, and mindfulness, you'll continually grow and refine your skills.

As you continue to evolve as a massage therapist, remember that learning is a lifelong journey. There's always something new to discover, and each person you work with will offer an opportunity to improve. Keep practicing, stay open to feedback, and trust your hands and instincts. The more you invest in your practice, the more capable you'll become at providing healing and relaxation to those you work with.

In the next chapter, we'll explore how to deal with common challenges that massage therapists face, including managing different client expectations, dealing with physical fatigue, and maintaining professional boundaries. But for now, take the time to reflect on your journey so far and continue honing your craft. Your journey toward becoming a master of massage is just beginning.

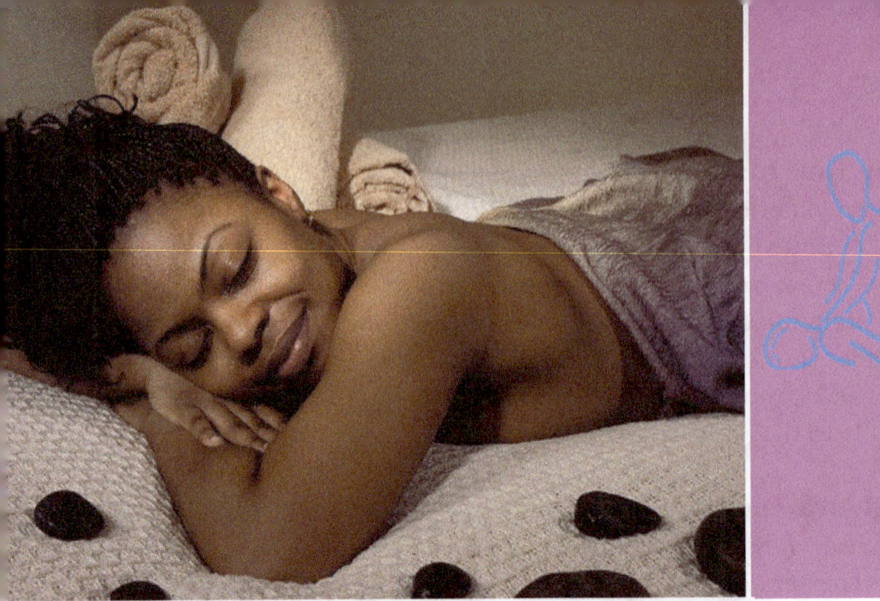

NAVIGATING COMMON CHALLENGES IN MASSAGE THERAPY

WHAT YOU'LL LEARN

- ◊ UNDERSTANDING AND MANAGING CLIENT EXPECTATIONS
- ◊ COPYING WTH PHYSICAL DEMANDS AND FATIGUE
- ◊ MAINTAINING PROFESSIONAL BOUNDARIES

Massage therapy is a fulfilling and transformative profession, offering the opportunity to enhance others' lives through healing touch. Yet, like all professions, it comes with its own set of challenges. Whether it's managing client expectations, dealing with the physical demands of the job, or maintaining clear professional boundaries, these challenges can sometimes feel overwhelming. However, with the right tools, mindset, and strategies, they can also serve as stepping stones to personal and professional growth.

In this chapter, we'll dive deep into how to navigate these common hurdles, equipping you with practical solutions and insights to thrive in your practice.

Understanding and Managing Client Expectations

Every client walks into a massage session with unique needs, goals, and expectations. Some may come for stress relief, others for chronic pain management, and a few might just be curious about trying something new. Your ability to identify and align with these expectations is crucial for creating a positive experience.

Listening and Setting the Stage

The first step in managing expectations is active listening. Begin each session with an open and friendly consultation. Use questions like:

- "What's the main reason you're here today?"

- "Are there any areas you'd like me to focus on?"

- "Do you prefer lighter or firmer pressure?"

This conversation not only helps you understand their goals but also builds trust and rapport. Let the client know what they can realistically expect from the session. For instance, if they're dealing with chronic pain, explain that while one session may bring some relief, ongoing treatments and lifestyle adjustments are often necessary for long-term improvement.

Navigating Unrealistic Expectations

Sometimes, clients may expect immediate results or have misconceptions about what massage therapy can achieve. In these cases, honesty is key. Frame the conversation around progress and collaboration:

- "While this session will help relax your muscles, deeper relief will likely require a few more treatments."

- "Massage is a great tool for pain management, but it works best alongside other healthy habits like stretching or exercise."

When faced with dissatisfaction, remain calm and professional. Use it as an opportunity to learn what they didn't enjoy and how you can improve. Most importantly, always leave the door open for constructive dialogue.

Coping with Physical Demands and Fatigue

Massage therapy is as physically demanding as it is rewarding. Long hours of standing, repetitive motions, and the physical effort required to deliver effective pressure can take a toll on your body. Without proper care, it's easy to experience fatigue, strain, or even injury.

Building Strength and Endurance

To maintain your physical health:

- Incorporate exercises like yoga, Pilates, or strength training to build muscle and flexibility.

- Focus on your core, as it provides stability and prevents back strain during sessions.

Stretching is also vital. Before and after your workday, dedicate time to stretch your arms, shoulders, back, and legs. These areas bear the brunt of your work and need regular care.

Maintaining Proper Ergonomics

Pay close attention to your posture during sessions. Position yourself so you can apply pressure using your body weight rather than relying solely on your hands. Keep your wrists straight, shoulders relaxed, and feet firmly grounded. Adjust the massage table height to prevent unnecessary bending or reaching.

Preventing Burnout

Massage therapy can also be emotionally draining. Balancing your schedule is critical. Avoid back-to-back sessions without breaks and ensure you're not overloading your day. Use downtime to recharge—whether that's enjoying a cup of tea, practicing mindfulness, or doing a quick stretch.

Remember, taking care of yourself isn't just for your benefit—it allows you to deliver the best possible care to your clients.

Maintaining Professional Boundaries

Boundaries are the foundation of a healthy therapist-client relationship. Without them, misunderstandings, discomfort, or even ethical breaches can arise.

Setting Clear Policies

At the outset, establish clear policies about session lengths, fees, cancellations, and the scope of your practice. Communicate these policies during the initial consultation or through written materials like a welcome packet or website.

Emotional Boundaries

While massage therapy can feel personal, it's essential to maintain a professional demeanor. Clients may share personal stories or emotions during a session, and while it's important to be empathetic, avoid becoming overly involved. A simple, "I hear you," or "That sounds challenging," can acknowledge their feelings without crossing into therapeutic territory.

Addressing Inappropriate Behavior

Occasionally, you may encounter clients who behave inappropriately, whether through suggestive comments or disrespectful actions. If this happens, address it calmly but firmly:

- "I want to ensure this is a safe and respectful environment for both of us. Let's refocus on the session."
If the behavior continues, don't hesitate to terminate the session. Protecting your boundaries is crucial for maintaining your professionalism and sense of safety.

Practical Solutions for Everyday Challenges

Massage therapy often involves juggling multiple responsibilities, from adapting techniques to meeting diverse client needs to managing your own energy levels.

- **Customizing Techniques:** Each client's body is unique. Use feedback to adjust pressure, tempo, and focus areas in real-time.

- **Efficient Scheduling:** Create a balanced schedule that avoids overworking yourself while ensuring consistent availability for your clients.

- **Staying Inspired:** Continuing education, whether through workshops or online courses, keeps your practice fresh and exciting. Learning new modalities or refining existing ones can reignite your passion.

Thriving in the Face of Challenges

Challenges are an inevitable part of any career, but in massage therapy, they can be opportunities for growth and learning. By addressing client expectations with honesty, protecting your physical health through self-care, and maintaining strong professional boundaries, you can navigate these challenges with confidence.

Always remember the incredible impact you have on others' lives. The relief, relaxation, and joy you bring to your clients make every challenge worthwhile. Embrace these hurdles as part of your journey, and let them shape you into a stronger, more compassionate practitioner. The rewards of massage therapy far outweigh its difficulties, and with the right approach, you can build a long-lasting and fulfilling career.

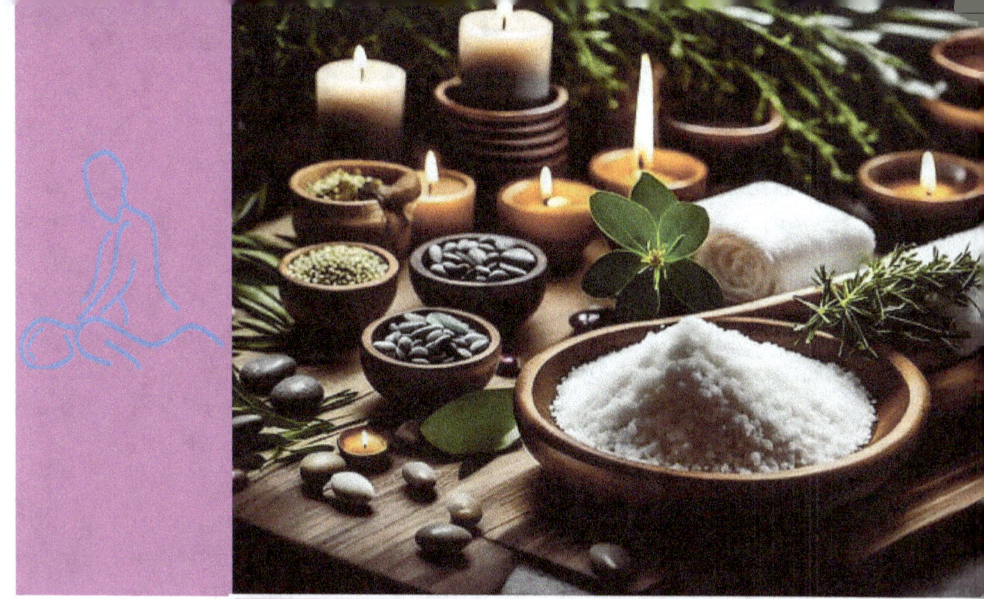

24

TAKING MASSAGE TO THE NEXT LEVEL

 **WHAT YOU'LL LEARN** 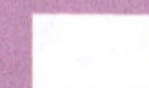

◇ EXPLORING OPPORTUNITIES IN MASSAGE THERAPY

◇ INTEGRATING MASSAGE INTO WELLNESS

Expanding Your Knowledge and Expertise

As your journey with massage continues, there may come a time when you feel ready to deepen your understanding and expand your skills. Massage is an evolving and dynamic field with a wide array of techniques, each offering unique benefits for both you and your clients. Whether you're aiming to enhance your personal practice or looking to grow your professional career, taking massage to the next level can open up new opportunities and increase your ability to help others.

In this chapter, we will explore the various opportunities in the professional field, and look at how you can integrate massage into a broader holistic wellness practice. From specialized massage methods to career expansion and cross-disciplinary collaboration, there are countless ways to refine your expertise and develop a practice that supports long-term growth.

Exploring Opportunities in Professional Massage Therapy

If you're considering taking massage to the next level, there are numerous opportunities for growth within the professional field. As a licensed massage therapist (LMT), your career can take many different directions, whether it's expanding your knowledge, specializing in niche areas, or exploring new professional settings. Let's take a closer look at the diverse opportunities available to you as you build your career.

1. Specialization and Certification:

One of the best ways to elevate your career is to specialize in certain types of massage therapy. Specialization allows you to cater to a particular client base and develop advanced skills in specific areas. Some common massage specialties include:

- **Sports Massage:** A technique tailored for athletes to address pre-event preparation, post-event recovery, and injury rehabilitation. Sports massage helps athletes maintain optimal performance and prevent injury.

- **Prenatal Massage:** Focuses on the unique needs of pregnant women. This type of massage can help alleviate the discomforts of pregnancy, such as back pain, swelling, and fatigue.

- **Craniosacral Therapy:** A gentle, hands-on technique that works with the craniosacral system (the membranes and fluid surrounding the brain and spinal cord) to release tension, promote relaxation, and improve overall well-being.

- **Reflexology:** Targets pressure points in the feet, hands, and ears that correspond to different organs and systems in the body. Reflexology can promote overall health and well-being by improving circulation and stimulating the body's natural healing processes.

By pursuing additional certifications and training in these or other specialized fields, you will deepen your expertise, attract more clients, and provide a broader range of therapeutic options.

2. Expanding Your Practice:

Once you've mastered a range of techniques and gained certification in various specialties, you might consider expanding your practice. There are many ways to grow and diversify your career. You could:

- **Open Your Own Practice:** If you prefer a more independent approach, consider opening a massage studio or wellness center. This allows you to create a personalized environment where you can offer your specialized services.

- **Mobile Massage Therapy:** Mobile massage therapy offers flexibility, as you travel to clients' homes or workplaces. This can be an excellent option for individuals who prefer the convenience of receiving massage in their own space.

- **Group Sessions and Workshops:** Hosting workshops or group massage sessions is another way to grow your business. You can teach self-care techniques or offer group relaxation sessions that promote wellness for multiple people at once.

Expanding your practice gives you the opportunity to work with more clients, offer a wider range of services, and build a reputation in your community as a trusted professional.

3. Collaborating with Other Health Professionals:

Massage therapy can complement many other healthcare practices, creating opportunities for collaboration. For example, many massage therapists work in conjunction with chiropractors, physical therapists, acupuncturists, and nutritionists. By partnering with these professionals, you can offer a more holistic treatment plan for clients and attract a diverse range of patients.

Being part of a multidisciplinary team allows you to provide integrated care, benefiting clients by addressing multiple aspects of their health at once. Additionally, cross-referrals between practitioners can help you build a stronger client base and expand your professional network.

Integrating Massage into a Broader Wellness Practice

As you grow in your massage practice, you may realize that massage is just one component of a broader wellness philosophy that supports long-term health and well-being. Integrating massage into a holistic wellness routine can enhance its benefits and create a more balanced approach to self-care.

1. Holistic Wellness Philosophy:

A holistic approach to wellness addresses the physical, emotional, mental, and spiritual aspects of health. Massage therapy fits seamlessly into this philosophy, as it not only relieves physical pain but also promotes emotional well-being by reducing stress and encouraging relaxation. By incorporating other wellness practices—such as healthy eating, yoga, mindfulness, and exercise—you can help clients achieve overall balance and health.

For example, yoga can increase flexibility, making muscles more receptive to therapeutic massage. Meditation and mindfulness help cultivate a sense of calm and awareness, which enhances the relaxation benefits of massage. Together, these practices can create a powerful synergy that promotes long-term wellness and personal growth.

2. Creating a Wellness Routine:

To truly take massage to the next level, you should encourage your clients to integrate massage into their broader wellness routine. Suggest creating a regular schedule for massages to manage stress, improve muscle recovery, and promote mental clarity. Encourage them to combine their massage sessions with other self-care habits, such as daily stretching, proper hydration, healthy eating, and regular physical activity.

By making massage part of a broader wellness plan, clients can experience lasting improvements in their health and well-being. Whether they're addressing chronic pain or simply seeking relaxation, massage becomes a cornerstone of their holistic health routine.

3. Cross-Disciplinary Collaboration:

As your massage practice evolves, consider collaborating with other health and wellness professionals. You could team up with personal trainers, life coaches, nutritionists, or therapists to offer a more comprehensive approach to well-being. A cross-disciplinary approach ensures that you are addressing all aspects of your clients' health, helping them create personalized care plans that lead to sustained, long-term benefits.

Final Tips for Confidence and Memorable Massages

Confidence in your ability grows with time, but here are some tips to keep you grounded and assured:

- **Trust Your Instincts:** Your intuition is a powerful tool. Listen to it, and let it guide your hands as you learn to sense what the body needs.

- **Focus on the Experience:** A memorable massage is more than just technique—it's about creating an atmosphere of care, calm, and connection.

- **Practice Self-Care:** Your hands, body, and energy are your greatest tools. Protect and nurture them by staying physically strong, mentally clear, and emotionally balanced.

- **Celebrate Your Progress:** Every massage you perform, every knot you ease, and every sigh of relief you hear is a milestone on your journey. Celebrate these moments as evidence of your growing mastery.

A Journey That Never Ends

Massage is a lifelong craft. It evolves with every person you work with, every technique you learn, and every challenge you overcome. Embrace this ever-changing journey with an open heart and a willingness to grow.

Remember, the true essence of massage lies not just in what you do but in how you make others feel. Through your hands, you offer healing, comfort, and a profound sense of care. That is your legacy as a massage practitioner.

As you continue on your path, know that mastery isn't about perfection—it's about passion, presence, and the courage to keep learning. Go forward with confidence, knowing that your touch has the power to transform lives, one massage at a time.

REFERENCES

16 types of massage ▮ Weald Chiropractic. (n.d.-c). Weald Chiropractic. https://www.wealdchiropractic.co.uk/what-are-the-16-different-types-of-massage/

Acche Vibes (acchevibes) - Profile | Pinterest. (2023, August 30). Pinterest. https://www.pinterest.com/acchevibes/

Cronkleton, E. (2023, August 31). What are the different types of massage? Healthline. https://www.healthline.com/health/types-of-massage

Stuart, A. (2023, August 2). Massage therapy styles and health benefits. WebMD. https://www.webmd.com/balance/massage-therapy-styles-and-health-benefits

MESSAGE OF THANKS

Thank you for taking the time to journey through this book. Massage is a beautiful way to connect with others, foster healing, and promote well-being. Every step you take, from learning a new stroke to helping someone feel better, is a step toward mastery.

Remember, this is just the beginning. Keep practicing, learning, and growing. The world needs your healing touch.

Warm regards,
Nicholas K. N.

www.ingramcontent.com/pod-product-compliance
Lightning Source LLC
Chambersburg PA
CBHW051559250726
48653CB00004BA/1226